DISCARD

Springer Series on the Teaching of Nursing

Diane O. McGivern, RN, PhD, FAAN, Series Editor
New York University Division of Nursing

Advisory Board: *Ellen Baer, PhD, RN, FAAN; Carla Mariano, EdD, RN; Janet A. Rodgers, PhD, RN, FAAN; Alice Adam Young, PhD, RN*

Jeanne M. Novotny, Ph.D., R.N., is the Frank Talbott, Jr. Visiting Professor at the University of Virginia. She was formerly Assistant Professor and Assistant Dean at the Frances Payne Bolton School of Nursing, Case Western Reserve University, Cleveland, Ohio; Associate Professor at the Vanderbilt University School of Nursing, Nashville, Tennessee; and Associate Professor at the Kent State University School of Nursing, Kent, Ohio. She received her B.S.N. from the Ohio State University; her M.S. in Nursing with a Clinical Specialty in Family Nursing from the Ohio State University; and her Ph.D. in curriculum and instruction in nursing with cognates in administration and international health from Kent State University. She is a member of the Ohio Nurses Association/American Nurses Association and Sigma Theta Tau.

Dr. Novotny has extensive experience with curriculum reform and program development. Her research interests are in the area of educational outcomes, distance learning, and determinants of success in nursing education programs on a national and international level. She has initiated a collaborative telecommunication course designed to prepare students to address the needs of culturally diverse patients through collaboration on research projects and clinical learning experiences. Dr. Novotny has served as a consultant to many national and international associations including Yonsei University, Seoul, Korea; University of Zimbabwe, Harare, Zimbabwe; and the Nursing Education Conference Planning Committees in Thailand and Brazil.

DISTANCE EDUCATION IN NURSING

Jeanne Novotny, PhD, RN
Editor

 Springer Series on the Teaching of Nursing

Springer Publishing Company, Inc.
536 Broadway
New York, NY 10012-3955

Acquisitions Editor: Ruth Chasek
Production Editor: Jeanne W. Libby
Cover design by James Scotto-Lavino

00 01 02 03 04 / 5 4 3 2 1

Library of Congress Cataloging-in-Publication Data

Distance education in nursing / Jeanne Novotny, editor.
    p.   cm.
    Includes bibliographical references and index.
    ISBN 0-8261-1341-9 (hardcover)
    1. Nursing—Study and teaching. 2. Distance education.
  I. Novotny, Jeanne.
    [DNLM: 1. Education, Nursing. 2. Education, Distance.
WY 18 D6138 2000]
RT73.D56 2000
610.73'071'1—dc21   00-020036
                                                CIP

Printed in the United States of America

Dedicated
to
My Parents

George Albert Lemire
and
Matilda Simon Lemire

Contents

Contributors

1. **Carolyn J. Bess, DSN, RN,** is an Associate Professor of Nursing and Director of the RN to MSN Program at Vanderbilt University School of Nursing. Her experience includes teaching and coordinating courses delivered in a variety of distance formats. She is also an expert in the learning needs of the working adult learner.

2. **Diane M. Billings, EdD, RN, FAAN,** is Professor of Nursing, Associate Dean for Teaching, Learning and Information Technologies, and Head of the Center for Teaching and Lifelong Learning at Indiana University School of Nursing. She has taught in and provided administrative leadership for distance education programs using written, video, audio, and Internet technologies. She is a distinguished authority and has published widely in the area of distance education. Her current research focuses on learner support and assessing the outcomes of web-based courses.

3. **Cecilia Campos, MPH, RN,** is Professor and Director of Research at the School of Nursing of the Catholic University of Chile. She is a member of the team of the Distance Learning Diploma Program on Nursing Leadership for Primary Health Care that is offered nationwide. She is host site coordinator of the Minority International Research Training Program directed by the College of Nursing of the University of Illinois. Her research, in collaboration with the University of Ottawa, Canada, focuses on health decisions of low-income women in Santiago, Chile.

4. **Karen L. Cobb, EdD, RN,** is Associate Professor and the Director of the Excellence in Teaching Center at Indiana University School of Nursing. She is a member of the faculty group involved in delivering nursing courses via the Internet. Her research focuses on assessment data related to students and the use of technology. She is the author of numerous articles and is co-author of a textbook on family nursing.

5. **Cornelia A. Corbett, MSN, RN, FNP,** is a clinician who is committed to distance learning. She is a preceptor for distance learning students and encourages the use of technology to promote community-based education. Her interest is in strengthening the relationship between education and practice.

6. **Eunice K. Ernst, CNM, MPH,** is the distinguished Mary Breckinridge Chair of Midwifery for the Frontier School of Midwifery and Family Nursing. As a practitioner, she served in a variety of capacities from public health nurse-midwife in the mountains of Kentucky to director of nurse-midwifery at Columbia Presbyterian Medical Center. She was also the Director of the National Association of Childbearing Centers. In 1989, after 10 years of planning, she founded the Community-Based Nurse-Midwifery Education Program of the Frontier School of Midwifery and continues to be a leader in bringing birth centers into the mainstream of health care delivery.

7. **Robert Gibson, MS,** is the Instructional Designer for the Wichita State University Media Resources Center in Wichita, Kansas. He is presently a doctoral student studying instructional technology and distance education through Nova Southeastern University in Fort Lauderdale, Florida. He developed the first completely Internet-delivered courses in the state of Kansas and serves as a web course designer for the faculty at Wichita State University.

8. **Sarah A. Hutchison, BSN, CCRN,** Nurse Manager of the Vanderbilt Trauma Center, is the nursing educator for the Trauma, Burn, Life Flight Patient Care Center. She is also an instructor in the Critical Care Program at the Vanderbilt University School of Nursing. Her interest is in distance technology as a way for employed nurses to maintain clinical competencies.

9. **Sonia Jaimovich, MPH, RN,** is Associate Professor of Nursing and Head of the Health Promotion and Self-Care Center at the Catholic University of Chile. She teaches Community Health Nursing in the undergraduate program and is a member of the team that develops courses using distance learning methodologies. Her research focuses on self-care and decision making in women.

10. **Stefanie J. Kelley, MSN, RN, CS, FNP,** is an Instructor of Nursing at the Frances Payne Bolton School of Nursing, Case Western Reserve

University. She has published and presented multiple papers on the topic of electronic technology and the Internet in advanced practice nursing. Her current teaching and research focuses on the use of electronic technology in the delivery of health promotion information to the general public.

11. **Joan E. King, PhD, RN, ANP, ACNP,** is Associate Professor and Director of the Acute Care Nurse Practitioner Program at Vanderbilt University School of Nursing. In addition to teaching, she maintains a clinical practice in the Pre-anesthesia Evaluation Clinic at the Vanderbilt Medical Center. Her current research focuses on hypothermia in trauma patients.

12. **Ilta Lange MSN, RN,** is Associate Professor and Director of the School of Nursing at the Catholic University of Chile. She teaches the Trends and Issues in Nursing Course that is offered to undergraduate students at Case Western Reserve University using distance education methods. She is a host site coordinator for the Minority International Research Training Program directed by the college of Nursing at the University of Illinois. She is well know in Latin America for her work in the development of a self-care nursing model which was implemented in primary care clinics in Chile and later incorporated throughout Latin America. She is one of the distinguished nursing leaders in South America.

13. **Judith M. Lewis, EdD, RN,** Professor of Nursing, has more than 20 years of experience in distance education for registered nurses seeking BSN and MSN degrees, including 9 years as director of the Statewide Nursing Program for California State University. Before the program added an on-line delivery system to reach nurses nationwide and around the world, a "semi-present" model with more than 200 teaching sites served a student population of 3,000 registered nurses across the state of California. Dr. Lewis created the Center of International Nursing Education at California State University, Dominguez Hills. Under her direction the Center has assisted countries in Latin America, Asia, Africa, and Europe to develop, implement, and evaluate no-tech, low-tech, and high-tech distance education programs for nurses. Her current research involves interviewing Chinese nurses in Beijing 12 years after they completed a distance education

program to determine what impact the program made on their professional practice. Dr. Lewis is CEO of the Claremont Consulting Group that provides consultation services to the national and international academic communities.

14. **Joan K. Magilvy, PhD, RN, FAAN,** is Professor and Director of the PhD Program at the University of Colorado Health Sciences Center School of Nursing in Denver, Colorado. She has been involved in all aspects of graduate nursing education. Recently, she led an extensive revision of the doctoral curriculum to increase access, flexibility, and use of multiple teaching-learning strategies. The focus of her research is rural aging and community-based health care services.

15. **Mary L. McHugh, PhD, RN, C, ARNP,** is an Associate Professor in the informatics track at the University of Colorado Health Sciences Center School of Nursing in Denver, Colorado. Formerly, she was the Chair of the American Nurses' Association Council on Computer Applications, and is a member of the Test Development Committee for Informatics Nursing Certification at the American Nurses Credentialing Center. She has received funding for nursing informatics research and has numerous publications in the field of nursing informatics and distance learning. She has developed and taught graduate courses using the Internet since 1996.

16. **Shirley M. Moore, PhD, RN,** is Associate Professor of Nursing at Case Western Reserve University, Cleveland, Ohio. She has a program of research that focuses on recovery following acute cardiac events. She has been an investigator on several federally funded projects evaluating the effects of computer-delivered nursing care on patient outcomes. She is interested in learning about ways to extend nurses into the lives of patients using non-face-to-face methods. She has written numerous articles on the use of computers to deliver nursing care.

17. **Carla L. Mueller, PhD(c), RN,** is Associate Professor of Nursing at the University of Saint Frances, Fort Wayne, Indiana. She is a certified web course facilitator. She has taught in distance education programs using print and audio technologies. She is a member of the Distributed Education Committee. Her current research focuses on

student experiences in the virtual classroom and assessing the outcomes of web-based courses.

18. **Jerry Murley, MEd,** is Assistant Professor and Director of Instructional Technology at the Vanderbilt University School of Nursing, Nashville, Tennessee. He is responsible for the administration, planning, and management of all learning resources. A veteran of project coordination, he has a particular interest in management, collaboration, and learning among multidisciplinary project team members who must use technology to work productively from various geographic locations.

19. **Julie C. Novak, DNSc, RN, CPNP,** is the Theresa A. Thomas Professor of Primary Care and Director of the Primary Care Nurse Practitioner Program at the University of Virginia. She is the project director of a distance learning grant funded by the Division of Nursing. Her research focuses on tobacco use prevention/cessation, and nurse practitioner practice and trends. She has published on a variety of child and family health promotion topics.

20. **Sandra W. Pepicello, PhD, RN,** is Dean of Nursing and Health Sciences at the University of Phoenix. In that role, she has administrative authority over one of the largest baccalaureate and higher degree nursing programs in the country. She has administered and taught in the distance education component that provides higher education for nurses throughout the world. Her research focus is on the education of working nurses and she has created rigorous and relevant programs for nurses in an era of changing health care.

21. **Susan D. Schaffer, PhD, FNP,** is Program Director for the Community-Based Family Nurse Practitioner Program at the Frontier School of Midwifery & Family Nursing, Hyden, Kentucky. She develops and teaches family nurse practitioner courses on interactive television and the Internet. Her research focus is on student outcomes.

22. **Marlaine C. Smith, PhD, RN,** is Associate Professor and Director of the Masters Degree Program at the University of Colorado Health Sciences Center School of Nursing. She taught outreach courses for graduate students across the state of Colorado from 1990-1996. She now teaches masters and doctoral nursing courses using interactive

video and participates in the development and evaluation of web-based courses in the curriculum. She is also the coordinator for the Mountain and Plains Project that is funded by Robert Wood Johnson.

23. **Susan E. Stone** is Program Director of the Community-Based Nurse-Midwifery Education Program at the Frontier School of Midwifery and Family Nursing, Hyden, Kentucky. This innovative, community-based, distance education program has graduated over 800 nurse-midwives since its inception in 1991. Her experience includes developing and teaching clinical courses to distance students, coordinating clinical sites for students at a distance, and partnering with other universities in the Delta Region to deliver midwifery education to rural areas. She is also coordinating the conversion of the current program to a web-based curriculum.

24. **Judith Sweeney, MSN, RN,** is Assistant Professor at the Vanderbilt University School of Nursing, Nashville, Tennessee. She has extensive experience in critical care nursing and directs the first year of the graduate program. Her research focus is on the outcomes of web-based courses for staff nurses in maintaining clinical competencies in physical and cardiac assessments.

25. **Lucille L. Travis, PhD, RN, CNA,** is Associate Dean and Associate Professor at Texas Woman's University. She is an expert in the evaluation of educational outcomes. Most recently, she has guided the implementation and evaluation of the revised doctoral and undergraduate curriculum at Texas Woman's University and incorporated the Internet and distance learning courses for the School of Nursing. Her current research focuses on tele-health research to examine the outcomes of heart failure patients utilizing home trans-telephonic symptom monitoring.

26. **Mila Urrutia, MSN, RN,** is Professor and Director of Graduate Affairs of the School of Nursing at the Catholic University of Chile. She teaches mental health and self-care nursing theory to students at the undergraduate level, in the nurse specialist program, and in continuing education courses. She is also the Distance Learning Director for the school. Her research focuses on educational outcomes using distance learning instructional strategies.

27. **Patricia Hinton Walker, PhD, FAAN,** is Dean and Professor at the University of Colorado Health Sciences Center, School of Nursing, Denver, Colorado. Previously, she served as the Kate Hanna Harvey Visiting Professor in Community Health at the Frances Payne Bolton School of Nursing at Case Western Reserve University, and was Associate Dean at both Emory University and the University of Rochester. Her research interests include cost and quality outcomes, interdisciplinary and advanced practice nursing, and the development of evidence-based care.

28. **JoAnn Zerwekh, EdD, RN, FNP, CS,** is Assistant Department Chair at the University of Phoenix, Tucson Campus and faculty at the Online Campus, Phoenix, Arizona. She teaches in the family nurse practitioner program and has extensive experience in distance education. She is the Executive Director of Nursing Education Consultants, Inc., Dallas, Texas. She is the author of numerous publications and works in various capacities as a consultant and nurse entrepreneur.

Foreword

I just came home from visiting Registered Nurses (RNs) who are enrolled in our distance education program, almost 300 miles from our main campus. These RN-BSN students were just finishing their second of three semesters with us. This second semester, like the past one, has been hard for them. They struggled to keep their sanity to "put it all together," that is, they worked full-time, they attended school full-time, while at the same time they tried to maintain some semblance of routine in their community and for their families. Besides taking on their additional content in our BSN program, they also had the value-added component of manipulating their courses via various forms of technology. These technology components included a syallweb, computer chats, video tapes, e-mails, bulletin boards, faxes, telephone discussions, and yes, sometimes the postal service. They have become astounded at all their flexibility, newly acquired active learning, and critical thinking skills.

Today, as they completed their semester coursework, they were tired, yet so enthusiastic, proud, and excited about all the educational material they had interacted with, still amazed that there is more to nursing than they had previously realized. They were so appreciative for the opportunity to enroll and interact with other distant RN colleagues from other rural, underserved areas. They spoke about how fortunate they were to have classes delivered to their homes so that they did not have to take the time to leave work and their community to travel to school. Many say that they could not have done it without the distance education opportunities. Additionally, they often spoke of their future (and immediate) goals to go on for some type of graduate education, which included specializing in anesthesia, midwifery, education, management, or becoming a nurse practitioner.

Not only are the students pleased, but so are their community leaders because they are "growing their own nursing leadership" with the advent of the web-based nursing program. Their nurses have the ability to stay in their community to further their education and thus, as the research has continually documented, these graduates will then stay in their community to use their new nursing education.

So why this long scenario? Simple. To me this scenario is the essence and passion of distance education. It is a steadfast commitment of providing accessible nursing education for life-long professional learning to "anyone, anytime." As you will learn in this book, effective learning takes place with effective instructional planning, no matter what methodology is used. The technology is only the vehicle or the messenger and during the education process, it should be relatively invisible to the learner.

Overall, Americans have come a long way with distance education in a short time. In less than 130 years, there has been an exciting evolution of strategies regarding distance education in the United States. It began in 1873 with correspondence courses which were sponsored by the Society to Encourage Studies at Home in Boston. This was followed by short courses and farmers' institutes by 1885. Then a commercial school for correspondence studies started in 1891. Radio was added to land grant college education by 1919 to broadcast short courses to constituents. The response to these early forms of distance education was strong, but unfortunately, drop-out rates were also high (65%). The lack of built-in faculty-student interactivity was thought to be the major problem.

Nursing also has had almost a century of work with distance education. The first documentation of nursing correspondence studies was in JAMA (1905), describing "an advertisement about correspondence studies in the latest issue of a respectable nursing publication stating, 'be a nurse, you can if you will." By 1913, another JAMA editorial said that this type of study for nurses "had had a remarkable growth in recent years." In 1923, correspondence courses were available for those nurses desiring public health education.

Nursing also became very creative with many of the telecommunications technologies. The University of Nebraska adapted a psychiatric nursing course for the telephone in 1956. By 1966, the University of Wisconsin had 24 telephone hookups with enrollments of 600 nurses. The rest of the technology movement with nursing education becomes a bit more familiar with video-based programs, satellite transmissions, mainframe programming, and computer-assisted instruction. Now, in a few short years during the 1990s, the advent of the Internet has produced an avalanche of users, stroking the keyboard to shop, to explore, to dialogue, and to learn.

But let's not kid ourselves—quantity does not mean ease. As any of these authors will tell you, effective distance education is hard, demanding work because it warrants taking the principles of effective interactive instruction and weaving it amongst the capabilities of the technology to produce an orchestration of educational activities that can be used by the student and faculty when they might be separated by time and space. The outcome of interactive learning is more intense for BOTH the faculty and the student.

Our whole nursing educational system, including faculty, student, and administrative activities, should be thoroughly reviewed. The techniques being done for distance education will eventually simply become traditional education. Distance education is not a sideline any longer, nor can we cop out saying that we are victims of our educational past, and "too mature" to change. Do we dare to hope that what we piece meal together will eventually form our future educational package for learning?

Hopefully, nursing will not become a cybercasualty by losing momentum as technology improvements continue. I see our two biggest personal challenges of the millennium as exemplary flexibility and willingness for creative change. While you may say that our future students will have more experience with computer technology, nursing still has a sizeable portion of providers without baccalaureate degrees who hopefully also will be our future students. How do we help students overcome the grieving process that happens as web-based courses shift their responsibility from passive to active learning?

Faculty, are you ready for on-line office hours, virtual student lounges, and cyber exams? How will nursing education add the multi-media look beyond the traditional clinical simulation center? Our nursing programs have typically been provided in linear, lockstep fashion, with virtually no student control. How fast can eager nursing students propel themselves through your educational program? How willing are you to develop partnerships among both public and private institutions to provide a myriad of student, library, and health care services? How can we accommodate accessibility to distance education for the handicapped student? With increasing web-based degree programs and course offerings and the idea of school catchment areas diminishing, how viable and differentiated will your courses and program be in our market-driven society?

Wow, these ideas are awesome, scary, and exciting as nursing becomes a part of the adept users of the cyberarena. Hopefully, nursing will continue to realize it needs to stay involved with the vision, while being challenged with all the opportunities AND questions inherent in any pioneering developmental process.

Myrna L. Armstrong, Ed.D., RN, FAAN
Professor and *staRNeTT Coordinator, School of Nursing
Texas Tech University Health Sciences Center
Lubbock, TX

Acknowledgments

I wish to acknowledge and express deep appreciation to Joyce J. Fitzpatrick, Elizabeth Brooks Ford Professor, Frances Payne Bolton School of Nursing, for her inspiration and motivation to achieve excellence; to Myrna L. Armstrong for her thought-provoking foreword; to Jeanette Lancaster, Dean, and Doris S. Greiner, Associate Dean, University of Virginia School of Nursing, for their commitment to nursing education and research; to Ruth Chasek, Nursing Editor, Springer Publishing Company, for her constant guidance; and to the two most wonderful men in the world, my husband, Bob, and my son, James.

Introduction

Jeanne M. Novotny

Nurses are assuming demanding professional responsibilities, related to technology, in the health care system. These responsibilities raise important questions about the application of technology in education, clinical practice, and research for all health care professionals. Electronic information has become a central component of the practice of nursing and represents a set of challenges that, although exciting and futuristic, often seems overwhelming and frustrating. Where are we headed and what do we want from the application of technology in our educational programs, practice sites, and research endeavors?

Every nurse has a part to play in the use of technology and must be familiar with the essentials of educational formats that depend on advanced information technology. The common goal for educators, practitioners, and researchers is to expand the frontiers of knowledge in the application of technology to advance nursing science. Technology is not the focus. Rather, the use of technology to access information and knowledge that was previously inaccessible is the focus.

This book is an attempt to present the complex technology of distance learning in nursing as it stands at this moment in time. It is intended for every nurse from the novice clinician to those in leadership positions. It addresses issues that cut across a wide spectrum of concerns related to distance learning. The focus is on the impact of technology on the way that we practice nursing and, in particular, the effect of technology on how students learn. The chapters in the book give a cross section of ideas from various nursing programs across the country, as well as basic how-to information for those who are thinking about applying some part of distance learning to their educational, clinical, and research endeavors. The authors of each chapter have explored the unique opportunities that exist for the nursing profession in the use of technology. They share their expertise and the exemplary models of their programs.

In Chapter 1, Judith Lewis outlines the fundamental essentials to consider when implementing a distance education program. Her knowledge of adult learning principles and her experience with the education of students at distance sites is key information for anyone wanting an overview of the state of the art of distance education. Chapter 2 is written by Mary McHugh and Rob Gibson and is filled with practical lessons for teaching on-line courses through the Internet. These two authors, in Chapter 3, go on to navigate us through the use of software tools for Web course development. Chapter 4, by Shirley Moore and Stefanie Kelley, describes the ways in which computer technology can enhance clinical learning. This chapter goes beyond the use of computers in the classroom and gives us examples of how to use technology in clinical situations. In Chapter 5, Carla Mueller and Diane Billings focus on the learner and nursing students. They discuss in detail the need for learner support in distance education courses and the strategies available to support learner success. Chapter 6 continues with Karen Cobb and once again, the expertise of Diane Billings, to provide us with a framework for assessing the learning outcomes of distance education.

Lucille Travis highlights, in Chapter 7, the juxtaposition of informatics with distance education and the use of technology as it relates to clinical practice. She describes the requirements for entry into practice and gives us an example of the essential course work needed for undergraduate students. In Chapter 8, JoAnn Zerwekh and Sandra Pepicello tell us about a program they have implemented at the University of Phoenix. This institution, which is the largest private accredited university for working adults, has had phenomenal success with distance education strategies that would have been unheard of a few years ago. Joan Magilvy and Marlaine Smith, in Chapter 9, present a second approach. They discuss the experiences and reflections of the University of Colorado distance graduate education program which delivers courses to rural, national, and international nursing student populations. Chapter 10, by Julie Novak and Diane Corbett, goes on to give us ideas about the preparation of primary care experts and a detailed plan of action for implementing distance education programs using interactive television.

Next follows an exciting chapter by Susan Stone, Kitty Ernst, and Susan Shaffer who describe activities underway at the Frontier Nursing Service. The Frontier Nursing Service has continued its historic mission of always being at the forefront of innovation by using a distance learning model for the education of nurse midwives. In Chapter 12, Carolyn Bess, an expert in RN to BSN education, discusses the redesign of the traditional program at Vanderbilt University and the movement of that program to the use of the Internet for course content delivery. Chapter 13, by Joan King, Jerry Murley, Sarah Hutchinson, Judith Sweeney, and Jeanne Novotny, discusses development of an on-line trauma course. The focus of this chapter is on the collaborative processes used between the School of Nursing and the Medical Center at Vanderbilt University.

Our international colleagues, Ilta Lange, Mila Urrutia, Sonia Jaimovich and Cecelia Campos, at the Catholic University of Chile in Santiago, describe their international projects and specifically the way in which two schools of nursing in two different countries used the Internet to teach a Trends and Issues in Nursing course. And, in Chapter 15, Patricia Hinton Walker examines the primary ways in which nursing is changing and concludes by giving us directions for the future.

This book presents some of the excellent distance education programs underway at several of the teaching institutions in the United States and elsewhere. The content will be useful to those interested in distance education opportunities and who wish to explore these and other programs to find one that best fits their needs. Hopefully, this book will give all nurses—educators, clinicians, and researchers—ideas about how to incorporate distance education principles into their lives and will foster the development of new knowledge for the discipline of nursing. This process will enhance both the learning of our students and the nursing care we deliver to our patients.

1

Distance Education Foundations

Judith M. Lewis

This chapter gives an overview of some essential considerations when planning and implementing a distance education program. The discussion is not exhaustive; the goal is to alert the reader to key elements and to stimulate further reading and consultation in those areas.

WHAT IS DISTANCE EDUCATION?

Embarking on an exploration of distance education is akin to entering the "erroneous zone." Misconceptions and misnomers abound. Many university teachers and administrators think that because they know general education and extension programs, they know distance education. Even after a thorough literature search, the waters may still be murky due to misunderstanding and to national differences. Garrison and Shale (1987) contend that a definition of distance education is akin to Jason's Fleece—tantalizing, much sought after, but ever elusive.

Although a distance education program may be described as nontraditional, not all nontraditional programs are distance education. An institution may extend its traditional programs to an off-campus location or remote site with the identical teaching-learning strategies used in course delivery on campus. These programs typically carry titles such as on-site, extension, off-campus, or outreach programs. Some of these programs also may be nontraditional by virtue of their use of different teaching-learning strategies, the addition of electronic technology, and/or modifications in the course delivery schedule. For example, there might be changes in the length of the class sessions or the interval between the class meetings to decrease travel costs (time and distance) for the teacher and/or student. If these programs were to be identified by using Scales's (1983) six types of distance education models, they would be categorized as Type VI—a fully supported program at a location geographically nearer the student than the parent institution is. The reality is that these programs are not distance education, yet they meet an educational need and are often the forerunner of an innovative distance education program (Lewis & Farrell, 1995).

Distance education has been broadly defined as a strategy in which the teacher or institution providing instruction is separated in either time or place, or both, from the learners (Moore, 1987). Other experts extend the definition to highlight the role of the academic institution, thus differentiating distance education from independent study. Holmberg (1986) describes distance education as study that is not under the continuous, immediate supervision of teachers present with their students on the same premises but that benefits from the planning, guidance, and teaching of a supporting organization. Burge and Lenskyi (1990) note that there is no physical space where teacher and class members come together and that distance education includes a variety of teaching methods planned and implemented by an institution. In accord with the following discussion, a broader description is warranted: A systematically planned adult learner–centered program is one in which integrated systems allow students to proceed in a self-directed manner, with few or no face-to-face meetings, toward achieving well-defined learning outcomes (Lewis & Farrell, 1995).

The American Council on Education (1996b) uses the term *distance learning* and describes it as a system and a process that connects learners with distributed learning resources. The council describes the separation, in place or time, between instructor and learner, among learners, and/or between learners and learning resources. The academic transaction occurs through one or more media, and the use of electronic media is not necessarily required. The offering institution is labeled the provider. It creates and facilitates the learning opportunity and has the responsibility to approve and monitor the quality of the learning experiences.

At times the term *open learning/open education* is used in conjunction with distance education. But distance education and open learning are distinct (Holmberg, 1986). Distance education refers mainly to mode of delivery; open education refers to *structural* changes that are permissive.

These changes are evident in the ideal open-learning environment described by Cunningham (1994) in which learners learn when they want to (timing, frequency, and duration) and how they want to (modes of learning). Further, learners are involved in their own assessment, negotiating criteria and methods by which assessment takes place, and in the process by which grading judgments are made. Students exert strong influence over academic policies and program operations.

Distance education may be open or closed. In the United States, distance education typically is closed, as the demands of the institution, regional accrediting bodies, and professional accrediting bodies tend to be prescriptive. Programs will have many of the structural characteristics attributed to open learning, but the institution and/or the faculty retain control of the content, course sequencing, and measurement of attainment of learning outcomes. These elements are seen as hallmarks of academic quality. Increased accessibility and flexibility are achieved through a variety of other strategies, including technology. As pioneering programs in distance education have demonstrated that their graduates are comparable to or exceed the qualifications of graduates of conventional programs, accrediting bodies have become more receptive to innovation in program delivery.

Distance education programs also are plagued by the use/misuse of a variety of descriptive terms: correspondence, open learning/open university, semi-present, independent study, assessment, and more recently, the electronic classroom. One common element is that little or no class (seat) time is required; the teacher and student may never meet face-to-face. The Carnegie unit determines academic equivalency: 45 hours of learning activities equal one semester credit. For example, a three-credit course offered on campus during a 15-week semester requires 3 hours of lecture per week and 6 hours of homework, for a total of 135 hours. The equivalency is met, and the course meets unit value transferability requirements between accredited institutions.

The Carnegie unit definition does not prescribe the nature of the learning activities. It is equally valid that all learning activities take place outside the traditional classroom. The classroom teacher never really knows how many hours a student actually engages in homework; instead, the teacher relies on performance outcomes to arrive at a grade. The same is true in distance education. Teachers prepare learning activities and assessments for each credit that, in their experience, they estimate will take the average student 45 hours to complete. This estimate can be verified through field testing in the formative phase of the program. Again, the student's performance on the course outcome measures determines the grade earned. Some programs keep no records of participation in learning activities; the emphasis is on the assessment of outcomes. The teaching-learning philosophy of such programs recognizes that the means of knowledge acquisition is not important, rather achievement—the demonstration of that knowledge through written and performance tests—is critical.

In an effort at clarification, some writers base distinctions among distance education programs on variables such as the use or nonuse of single, multiple, or integrated technologies; the degree of learner independence as opposed to the need for more support; and the extent of geographical separation (Faibisoff & Willis, 1987; Romiszowski, 1993). But as the preceding discussion reveals, distinctions may not be clear, and definitions may be blurred. Regional, national, and international customs add their own influence. It is important to proceed with a common understanding when a faculty is developing a distance education program or disseminating information about it.

MAXIMIZING THE POTENTIAL OF DISTANCE EDUCATION

The competitive environment of today, combined with the herd mentality to get on the technology bandwagon, means that many educators and institutions are busy trying to replicate the traditional classroom electronically. This approach assumes that distance education equates with technology and that traditional practices using technology are best. Another term has been coined—*distributed education*. This term assuages those who previously decried distance education but now that bells, whistles, and funding are available, want to be involved. And supposedly, this new term distinguishes it from the negative connotations, warranted or not, that some attribute to distance education; but again, it will likely add to the confusion on terms.

Developing and implementing a quality distance education program to serve off-campus students should not be undertaken haphazardly. The planners require knowledge of teaching and learning and the target student population, as well as knowledge of the discipline. Further, they must be creative thinkers to elaborate and convey the vision and diligent managers in the development of the necessary systems and subsystems. The hard work in distance education occurs before students are ever admitted. For example, in the area of student support, Feasley (1983) describes the many elements that should be considered in that system alone. The effort put into developing a seamless program with quality learning materials, a sound curriculum-delivery system, and strong communication channels is rewarded later when the satisfying student-teacher interaction is the prominent faculty role.

The spirit and potential of distance education can best be realized by programs that are specifically designed and implemented on the basis of the needs of the identified population of learners for whom the program is intended (Lewis & Farrell, 1995). The focus of the program is student learning rather than presentation of information. The curriculum is competency-based, prior learning is assessed and validated, and skills to promote each student's success are developed. The role of the teacher is that of facilitator and collaborator in the learning process rather than giver of information. The student is seen as a proven learner who brings a wealth of resources to the academic environment.

ADULT LEARNING PRINCIPLES

In distance education programs, students may be of any age, and the program of study may be for personal enrichment only or lead to a recognized certificate, a diploma, or a degree. However, the typical target audience is adults at the high school or college level. Even so, the program may or may not be based on adult learning principles. For collegiate-level programs, particularly for nursing, the inherent nature of a program based on adult learning principles promotes lifelong learning and fosters the development of leadership skills. In nursing, distance education is most often a BSN completion program or graduate-level program. There are basic programs that make some courses available at a distance, but whether there will ever be a generic distance education BSN program is for the future to reveal.

When experienced nurses return to school for further formal education, they respond extremely well to a program that is "androgogical" rather than pedagogical if they receive appropriate support. This is true even if their prior experience has been in a pedagogical model. An effective strategy to promote this positive response is to offer an initial course that introduces the student to the program's teaching-learning philosophy, the new roles of the teacher and learner, and provides practical experience with the learning modalities and the student behaviors that underpin success in the program. The teaching-learning philosophy and the learning activities should reflect adult developmental considerations.

Assumptions About the Development of Adult Learners

- They have moved from viewing themselves as dependent to viewing themselves as self-directed human beings.
- The have accumulated a growing reservoir of experience that becomes an increasing source for learning.
- Their readiness to learn has become increasingly influenced by the developmental tasks of their social roles.
- Their perspective has changed from postponed application of knowledge to immediate application, and they are particularly interested in how knowledge they acquire can be applicable to real life (Knowles, 1975).

In androgogy, a term introduced by Malcolm Knowles (1980) to distinguish between the learning needs of adults and those of children (pedagogy), the central theme is that the student is a capable decision maker and is an active participant rather than a passive recipient in the teaching-learning process. Teachers in the program must be oriented to their responsibilities as well. They need to recognize the value of a less hierarchical learning environment and embrace the role of facilitator-guide to vivify an adult learning environment.

Assumptions About the Learning Environment

Pedadogy	Androgogy
The climate is authoritative.	The climate is relaxed and informal.
Competition is encouraged.	Collaboration is encouraged.
Teacher sets goals.	Teacher and class set goals.
Decisions by teacher	Decisions by students and teacher
Lecture by teacher	Process activities and inquiry projects
Evaluation by teacher	Evaluation by teacher, self, peers
Teacher-directed	Self-directed

One of the most important contributions of androgogical theory (Knowles, 1975) was to increase awareness of the learner's rightful place at the center of the instructional process. The perception of the learner as an active participant in this process affects the choice of program delivery methods and instructional strategies. Recognizing that adults are capable of self-direction can have a significant impact on the teaching-learning process and the roles traditionally fulfilled by the teacher and student.

In all areas of assessment every student is able to achieve an A or an F. Grading is never done on the curve. Adult learner–centered programs are competency-based, and the student faces only self-competition against a set of criteria (established by the faculty) with the minimum acceptable achievement level. Performance expectations are fully elaborated—students do not have to spend time trying to discover what is expected. There is consistency in grading among faculty members teaching the same course regardless of where the student resides.

Viewing students as adult learners affects the curriculum as well as the teaching-learning process, and in fact, the two components are deliberately melded. For example, because a student's prior learning is valued, repetitive content is avoided; because the adult student is self-directed, assessment rather than course enrollment is an option. Within a course, the learning contract can be used to capitalize on the student's self-directedness, prior learning, and experience.

Learning contracts allow students to select their own time and place for application of their new knowledge and skill. This strategy is particularly appropriate for registered nurses in clinical courses. The setting is not critical; rather, it is the availability of desired learning experiences and a preceptor to assist the student to access those experiences that are essential. Per current accreditation expectations, the BSN program produces a generalist. This is disappointing to some registered nurses. However, when the program does not dictate the clinical site, there are many options available. For example, a student interested in care of the neonate can elect to do leadership and management clinical courses in the neonatal setting. In caring for families in the community, the caseload would include families with newborns. And of course, a research or change agentry project would be in an area of the student's choice.

A concern detected by Liners and Hrobsky (1996) is a lack of clarity among preceptors and students regarding expectations. The contract form is not magical nor elaborate, yet it lends structured clarity to the precept-ored learning experience. A simple three-column format is effective.

Objectives	Learning Activities	Evidence of Achievement

Courses will have prescribed outcome objectives, which are entered in column 1. But the course may be tailored. For example, in a leadership or management course, a student who is an experienced head nurse may want to write higher level objectives that subsume the prescribed ones. In this way, the nurse's clinical time is not repetitive but builds on his or her prior knowledge and experience. And this strategy recognizes that a registered nurse has different needs from those of a generic student (Andrusyszyn & Maltby, 1993).

Students also write their complementary objectives in column 1, show-ing the relationship to the subsumed objectives. This allows the student to explore in more depth an area of interest that coincides with the overall goals of the course. Whereas each student is held accountable for achieving the objectives at a prescribed level, column 2 will be different for different students. The identified learning activities reflect the particular practice setting, the student's background, and the student's interest. This is where the student is self-directed in identifying what she or he needs to achieve the objectives. Column 3 lists the prescribed course evaluation measures and student-generated measures, and by virtue of the order of presentation, the relationship between objectives and measurement of outcomes is evi-dent. The course professor, the preceptor, and the student are all signatories to the student-generated learning contract.

Because the program capitalizes on the assets that the employed adult brings to the educational setting, the workplace becomes a laboratory, whether or not it serves as a clinical course setting. The student in the employee role sees the immediate application of new knowledge to real problems encountered at work or in other settings or other roles (Knowles, 1986). Teachers who make use of these actual problems within the academic transaction vivify theory-based practice, promote higher order thinking, and boost the confidence of the student in problem identification and problem solving.

In teaching students how to prepare their own learning contracts, the process is made analogous to that of the nursing process—only this time the nurse herself is at the center. Sometimes students are reluctant to make their own academic decisions. Even nurses who make critical decisions about their patients or their practice setting every day may be hesitant. They often come from varied pedagogical backgrounds. For this reason, an initial course that introduces students to an adult learner–centered program and the new roles of the teacher and student is a wise investment. Such a course should expose the students to the theory and practices underlying the program in a nonthreatening environment. This makes returning to school a more satisfying experience and increases the likelihood of success.

THE ACADEMIC TRANSACTION

In many education settings the emphasis is on giving information and then testing recall through midterm and final examinations, but the emphasis should be placed on the academic transaction. The transaction is actually a dialogue (academic conversation) between student and teacher, in which raw information is transformed into knowledge through negotiation of meaning. Traditionally, the academic transaction occurs simultaneously with information giving in the classroom. In the typical classroom the teacher lectures for an hour and then asks, "Are there any questions?" Depending on the amount of time remaining, the assertiveness of individual students, and the size of the class, the academic transaction takes place—at least for some students. Office hours are another opportunity for the academic transaction; again, if the student is assertive, an appointment is available and the professor actually appears.

Distance education approaches the academic transaction from another perspective. The teacher is not involved in directly giving information to the student. Instead, the teacher or a team of teachers (often with the assistance of instructional design experts) prepares the learning materials, which contain information and learning activities and direct the student to additional resources. The provision of information through these learning materials takes place separately from the academic transaction. The materials usually are in print format but also may be audiovisual or electronic, and they reach the student by whatever delivery system the program is using. The learning activities embedded in these materials require students to respond to the information, to think about their thinking (metacognition), and to confer with other students; and they provide built-in opportunities to interact individually and in small groups with the professor—the academic transaction.

In distance education the academic transaction may be high-tech or low-tech, and it may be synchronous (student at a distance receiving course at the same time it is being taught) or asynchronous (student can access course at own convenience). A distance education program can be solely based on correspondence—low-tech and asynchronous—and be of high academic quality. The University of Chicago is credited with offering the first U.S. correspondence course in 1890, followed by the University of Wisconsin in 1896. The U.S. military has long provided correspondence courses to members of the armed forces. When telephones became ubiquitous, they were added to the communications armamentarium. With the current availability of affordable technology, bidirectional communication now takes place through the postal service, phone, fax, E-mail, teleconferencing, chat rooms, and threaded discussions. Synchronicity decreases flexibility and an asynchronous academic transaction is just as effective. The use of technology and whether it is synchronous or asynchronous are not the distinguishing elements (Russell, 1998). The technology extends the reach of education to previously unserved or underserved populations as well as to those who prefer a more self-directed learning environment. Therefore, a decision to require all students to be on-line, or in a teleconference, or in a classroom at the same time should be carefully considered.

Many programs use technology singly or in combinations. The nursing programs at California State University, Dominguez Hills, have always been offered as distance education, beginning with some face-to-face meetings, moving to video supported by E-mail, and now evolving as fully Web-based (Johnston & Lewis, 1995). Pennsylvania State University has long offered distance education programs and has been a pioneer in technology for program delivery. Touro University International, the distance education arm of Touro University, offers degrees totally on-line. Students around the world can apply, pay fees, and complete courses solely through the Internet. The Web-based courses include threaded discussion and video and audio streaming. Synchronous computer conferencing (voice and video) is offered as an option; the teacher is available and the student participates as desired. Students working in small groups determine their own need for synchronous on-line conferencing among themselves.

The academic transaction reveals to the professor whether or not the student understands. Sometimes in typical classrooms the revealing is only through the examination, as there is little time to interact individually with every student. A satisfying aspect of distance education is that students can no longer avail themselves of academic camouflage—hiding out in the crowd, outwaiting the clock, or relying on a more assertive student to pose the questions arising in their own thinking. Because the information-giving aspect of teaching has already been accomplished, the professor's course time is dedicated to assessment and the academic transaction. The teaching-learning process includes scheduled interchange between the teacher and the student and spontaneous conversations initiated by either the student or the teacher. A well-designed distance education program requires every student to respond and to take a leadership role in his or her own learning, in small-group work and in other learning activities.

The scary aspect of the teacher role from a professor's viewpoint is that she or he can no longer rely on prepared notes to fill the class time. Not only must the professor be master of the content but also an effective discerner and someone who can develop a rapport with students who are not physically present. Teaching strengths must include assisting students in the metacognition process, drawing parallels, bridging theory and practice, and promoting the student's higher order thinking capabilities. Some teachers have these skills; others can be helped to develop them—they are valued in any academic program; they are essential to quality distance education.

INSTRUCTIONAL DESIGN

Just as there is a science of education, there is the technology of instructional design—the application of the science to practice. The development of learning materials for a particular target audience requires knowledge and skill beyond that of the typical teacher. High-quality materials are the expected outcome when experts from the discipline work with those that hold master's and doctoral degrees in instructional design.

Nursing has an advantage over many other professions and disciplines. Accreditation expectations have encouraged nursing programs to have a coherent curriculum with clearly articulated outcomes. Nurse educators are accustomed to behavioral objectives and performance outcomes from their academic role and from their clinical practice role. The faculty's philosophy of nursing and of teaching and learning form the foundation of the instructional design process. Nurse educators bring to the instructional design and development process their knowledge of the discipline and the practice setting, their knowledge of the target audience, and their years of teaching experience. Instructional designers bring in-depth knowledge of how people learn; teaching strategies that harmonize with cognitive, affective, and psychomotor learning processes; and a gamut of learning activities—from no tech to high-tech—that recognize a range of learning styles, encourage higher order thinking, and promote student attainment of the learning outcomes. They also bring expertise in a variety of evaluation measures, student assessment, and formative and summative evaluation of learning materials and processes.

In forming a team it is important to have the right people. A common error is thinking that all one needs to do Web-based instruction is a webmaster to "mount" the course. The typical webmaster is not a qualified instructional designer but a technical expert who plays an important role on the team. Another error is the independent development of each course. First, the team has to make some decisions that will affect all courses. These include the visual appearance of the materials, the format and sequence, and the chunking and structuring of information. Be aware that instructional design had its earliest applications in business and industry, so care must be taken that materials do not appear too "industrial" or "masculine." Consistency is a stress reducer; students should not have to expend energy becoming acquainted with many different formats in one curriculum. However, consistency does not negate creativity. Materials should be gender-neutral, and fonts, type size, colors, diagrams, feedback loops, and sophistication of language should be responsive to the student audience. A tool developed by Lewis (1998) is useful in assessing print learning materials for a distance education program. In addition to the conventional descriptors for print materials, the tool addresses the academic transaction and the program's curriculum-organizing framework,

The preparatory phase of the program, when instructional design, development, and program delivery decisions are made, is crucial. When students have access to a program of planned instruction, where the course materials are systematically designed and provide direction to additional resources, they can proceed in a self-directed manner and be successful in meeting the specified outcomes for each course.

EVALUATION OF DISTANCE EDUCATION PROGRAMS

Because distance education is education, the evaluation process differs little from that undertaken for traditional programs. For example, the following indicators, adapted from Paul (1990), are usually applied when considering conventional and unconventional programs:

Completion rates: the proportion of learners who complete the courses in which they are registered

Graduation rates: the proportion of learners who obtain the academic credentials they seek

Persistence rates: the proportion of learners who are eligible for and take another course

Measures of cost: the cost per course, per completion, and per graduate

Although the modern era of distance education in the United States goes back more than 20 years, the various forms of distance education program delivery are still viewed as new or untested by many within and external to academia. And, since the teaching-learning process does not take place behind the closed classroom door and the learning materials are generally available, distance education is more open to scrutiny. Detractors review materials with a magnifying glass, students often have a high degree of sophistication, and among the public-at-large, there is a tendency to judge print, video, and web pages against Madison Avenue standards. Learning materials produced by the program must be well produced and accurate. As noted on the following list, adapted from Gooler (1979), program materials as well as the program's organization and societal contribution are among the indicators for distance education quality.

Access: the proportion of learners who complete courses in which they are registered

Relevancy: to what extent is the program relevant to national, local, and individual needs?

Quality: Is the graduate effective in her or his new role?

Learning materials: Are the materials current and appropriately presented for target learners?

Seamlessness: How well do the various systems and subsystems interrelate and function?

Learner outcomes: To what extent do learners achieve program outcome competencies? To what degree do they meet their own goals? Are there any unanticipated outcomes?

Impact: How does the program affect society, other programs, and institutions?

Generation of knowledge: To what degree does the program contribute to the body of knowledge about adult distance education?

The American Council on Education (1996a) compares outcome achievement between learners at a distance and learners exposed to traditional classroom lecture methods. In particular, they question whether the technology helps the learner achieve the learning outcomes. Seven categories—learning design, learning objectives and outcomes, learning materials, technology, learner support, organizational commitment, and subject—are included in the evaluation criteria. Key questions within each category stimulate inquiry into essential elements to evaluate.

Two other indicators, identified by Paul (1990) as essential to any program evaluation plan but more difficult to measure, are skill development and postgraduate performance. The latter coincides with several of the indicators listed above. The former, skill development, refers to the degree to which learners develop self-directed learning skills and take responsibility for their own learning. Because these student behaviors are inherent in an adult learner–centered distance education program, the graduates of such programs should highly reflect this ability.

When planning for any educational program, it is important to know where you want to go before you finalize your plans for how to get there. Designing the formative and summative evaluation processes should coincide with program development. It means discovering the ways to know, with little or no doubt, that the program goals have been achieved.

Evaluation processes are the means by which the academic legitimacy of an innovative program is established and external accreditation is earned.

WHY DISTANCE EDUCATION?

Higher education is changing, and the changes go to the philosophical core of how one teaches, the relationship between teacher and student, the way in which a class is structured, and the nature of the curriculum. The paradigm of higher education is changing, becoming more learner-centered. Distance education has already embraced this paradigm— perhaps even initiated it with those programs that emphasize adult learning.

Access to higher education for the average person began in the United States following World War II, when college benefits were made available to returning veterans. Over time, enrollment of women increased though no special government funding allocation was made. This issue of equity had great significance for nursing. Historically, women did not enjoy equal access to American higher education. And even today, with the multiple roles women fulfill in our society (Green, 1987), academically capable nurses often find it challenging to enter and complete a traditional university program.

In 1965, the American Nurses Association (ANA) defined the minimum academic preparation for entry into the practice of professional nursing as the baccalaureate level. Needless to say, there was a great deal of frustration among nurses; a desirable societal goal was established, yet reasonable means for nurses to achieve that goal were not readily available (Lewis & Cobin, 1985). Campus-based traditional programs that developed RN tracks and second step programs (BSN completion) were important changes, but it wasn't until distance education was made available to nurses that significant progress was made. The very existence of these BSN completion programs made the ANA goal an achievable personal goal for many nurses.

National studies have predicted the need for more advanced practice nurses. Again, distance education is responding to the need with a variety of programs. Although graduate-level degree programs are not as prevalent as those for undergraduates, there are opportunities for nurses to become practitioners, teachers, clinical specialists, and administrators through distance education programs. An example is the Regents College of New York, which offers an MSN in clinical systems management. The degree uses a combination of course-delivery methods: self-paced learning modules, each with a terminal assessment; preceptorial courses; and courses with required on-line discussion components. A variety of support services are available on-line.

MAINSTREAMING DISTANCE EDUCATION

Past experience shows that the most successful distance education programs are housed in institutions dedicated to that purpose. One reason is that the function of distance education is different from and more complex than that of most conventional programs (Keegan, 1993). To be cost-effective, distance education relies on economy of scale, and there is an interrelationship between logistics, organization, costs, and educational issues. There are multiple systems and subsystems that must be well managed (Murgatroyd & Woudstra, 1990). Some of these systems are extensions of regular university processes, some are parallel systems, and others are unique to distance education. A business model for program operations is appropriate—one in which the student/consumer is central, and operations are seamless and lean. All program personnel are consumer-oriented, and teachers usually wear more than one hat—for example, member of course design team, recruiter, and on-line facilitator. And all personnel are familiar with the various systems and subsystems, recognizing their interrelatedness and the importance of avoiding unilateral changes. Many of these elements may be given only lip service in the conventional institution; they may even be seen as an anathema.

In the traditional university distance education may be viewed as a less desirable alternative and not really an integral part of the university's mission—a program to be tolerated, not nurtured. Because students reside around the state, the nation, and the world, they do not make a visual impact on campus. Distance education teachers may not be equitably recognized in the usual retention, tenure, and promotion processes and are unofficially considered "second class" in the university pecking order. The philosophy of the adult learner as a client and the need to make certain services available to off-campus students take second place or are ignored.

However, times are changing. Student enrollment in distance education programs is growing, including fields such as engineering, information technology, library science, and mathematics. Another example is nursing.

In 1981 the United States had one nursing program that was assessment only (Regents College) and one statewide distance education BSN completion program (California State University). Today registered nurses have many choices for earning a BSN. It is predicted that the number of graduate programs will increase on an ever steeper trajectory as more students seek master's and doctoral degrees and as graduates of the many BSN-completion distance education programs seek a similar learning environment for their next higher education endeavor. Once students feel the personal empowerment and sense of responsibility and accomplishment gained in an androgogical environment, they find a more pedagogical setting stifling and demeaning.

The academic quality and legitimacy of well-designed and -executed distance education programs has been proved. There is already evidence that teachers who explore distance education with an open mind find useful strategies to take back to the traditional classroom. Many find working with adult learners in distance education so enjoyable that they don't return to their previous teaching assignment. Parity between distance education and education in general has been an issue (Jevons, 1984). The lack of clarity in terminology and the tendency of some academicians to make assumptions did not help. But as cross-pollination occurs, distance education will no longer have to seek "parity of esteem," as it will have parity by virtue of what it is—education (Garrison & Shale, 1987). The digital revolution has profoundly altered previous limitations of time and space, and distance education is emerging as part of mainstream education (American Council on Education, 1996b). All disciplines should be attentive to the needs of the learning society. Nursing can continue to be at the cutting edge and through innovative education move the profession toward its goals for practitioners and for the society it serves.

REFERENCES

American Council on Education, Center for Adult Learning and Educational Credentials. (1996a). *Distance learning evaluation guide*. Washington, DC: ACE Central Services.

American Council on Education, Center for Adult Learning and Educational Credentials. (1996b). *Guiding principles for distance learning in a learning society*. Washington, DC: ACE Central Services.

Andrusyszyn, M. A., & Maltby, H. R. (1993). Building on strengths through preceptorships. *Nurse Educator Today, 13*(4), 277–281.

Burge, E., & Lenskyi, H. (1990). Women in distance education: Issues and principles. *Journal of Distance Education, 5*(1), 30–37.

Cunningham, I. (1994). *The wisdom of strategic learning: The self-managed learning solution.* London: McGraw-Hill.

Faibisoff, S. G., & Willis, D. J. (1987). Distance education: Definition and overview. *Journal of Education for Library and Information Science, 27,* 223–232.

Feasley, C. E. (1983). Serving learners at a distance: A guide to programs and practice. In *ERIC Higher Education Research Report*, No. 5. Washington, DC: Association for the Study of Higher Education.

Garrison, D. R., & Shale, D. (1987). Mapping the boundaries of distance education: Problems in defining the field. *American Journal of Distance Education, 1*(1), 7–13.

Gooler, D. D. (1979). Evaluating distance education programmes. *Canadian Journal of University Continuing Education, 6*(1), 43–55.

Green, C. P. (1987). Multiple role women: The real world of the mature RN learner. *Journal of Nursing Education, 26*(7), 266–271.

Holmberg, B. (1986). *Growth and structure of distance education.* London: Croom Helm.

Jevons, F. (1984). Distance education in a mixed institution: Working toward parity. *Distance Education, 5*(1), 24–37.

Johnston, K., & Lewis, J. (1995). Reaching RNs through the electronic classroom. *Nursing and Health Care,* 237–238.

Keegan, D. (1993). *Theoretical principles of distance education.* London: Routlege.

Knowles, M. S. (1975). *Self-directed learning. A guide for learner and teachers.* Englewood Cliffs, NJ: Cambridge Adult Education.

Knowles, M. (1980). *The modern practice of adult education: From pedagogy to androgogy* (rev. ed.). Chicago: Follett.

Knowles, M. S. (1986). *Using learning contracts: Practical approaches to individualizing and structuring learning.* San Francisco: Jossey-Bass.

Lewis, J. M., & Cobin, J. T. (1985). Mediated learning: A new pathway to the BSN. In J. C. McCloskey & H. K. Grace (Eds.), *Current issues in nursing* (2nd ed., pp. 257–268). Boston: Blackwell Scientific.

Lewis, J. M., & Farrell, M. (1995, June). Distance education: A strategy for leadership development. *Nursing and Health Care,* 184–187.

Lewis, J. (1998). An evaluation tool for print-based interactive learning materials. *Proceedings of the Institute for Innovation in Education.* Belo Horizonte, Brazil: Federal University of Minas Gerais.

Liners, K. A. L., & Hrobsky, P. E. (1996). Use of clinical map guidelines in precepted clinical experiences. *Nurse Educator, 21*(6), 19–22.

Moore, M. G. (1987, September). University distance education of adults. *Tech-Trends*, 13–18.

Murgatroyd, S., & Woudstra, A. (1990). Issues in the management of distance education. In M. G. Moore (Ed.), *Contemporary issues in American distance education* (pp. 44–57). New York: Pergamon.

Paul, R. H. (1990). *Open learning and open management.* New York: Nichols.

Romiszowski, A. (1993). *Telecommunications and distance education.* Syracuse, NY: Syracuse University.

Russell, T. L. (1998). *No significant difference: Phenomenon as reported in 248 research reports, summaries, and papers* (4th ed.). Raleigh: North Carolina State University.

Scales, K. (1983, November). A typology applied to distance education in British Colombia. *Lifelong Learning, 7*(3), 14, 26–28.

2

Teaching a Web-based Course: Lessons From the Front

Mary L. McHugh and Robert Gibson

More and more universities, colleges, and community colleges are listing "expansion of our Web-based course offerings" as one of their strategic objectives for the year 2000 and beyond. These authors predict that, by the year 2010, most universities will offer at least some of their degree programs as Web-based, distance education options. Although the number of students pursuing higher educational offerings will almost certainly increase, the proportion of students who are able to live on or near campus and attend school full-time will almost certainly decrease. The reality is that the major growth in demand for higher education is from people who are employed full-time, have families, and must fit their schoolwork around the demands of employment and family life. Institutions of higher education that choose to ignore the changes in the profile of the university's customer population and the increasing demand by adults for education that fits their schedules may well find themselves forced to downsize.

This chapter is written for those members of university instructional communities who are interested in focusing more energy in teaching online courses through the Internet. It will address the differences among traditional, correspondence, and Web-based modalities for teaching undergraduate and graduate courses. Strengths and limitations of each modality will be addressed. Techniques of developing and implementing a Web-based course and degrees through the Web, with special emphasis on how to adapt teaching methods to the Internet, will be discussed. Techniques that have proved unsuccessful will be presented, as well as tips for success.

KEY DEFINITIONS: THE NATURE OF THE BEAST

A *traditional on-campus course* is defined as a course in which students attend class in a university classroom one or more times per week, purchase their text materials at the university bookstore, and receive paper handouts in class from the instructor. Study guides may be purchased or made available in learning labs on campus. The student-instructor interaction is either face-to-face or via telephone. Often, students have group projects for which they schedule themselves during their out-of-class time. Students have access to the books, journals, and other materials in the on-campus library and for a fee can obtain other materials through interlibrary loan. Traditionally, on-campus courses make the assumption that some students may not have access to the Internet, and the course can be successfully completed without that access.

A *correspondence course* is defined as a course in which there is no on-campus requirement. The student pays a single fee for tuition, books, and supportive materials. Usually, the student must independently study the materials, schedule exams, and mail the exams back to the college or university for grading. When the student completes all requirements, a grade is sent. That is, there may or may not be any provision for communication between students and faculty, such as through mail or telephone calls. Typically, there is a final deadline for completion of all requirements, but the deadline is usually generous, and students may learn at their own pace.

A *Web-supported course* is a traditional on-campus course in which students have access to all the resources listed above. In addition, the course instructor places some materials on the Internet for students to use and perhaps copy if they wish. Such materials as the course syllabus, study guides, assignment guides, grading criteria, lecture notes, and/or slide presentations from the class lectures may be made available to students at the class Internet site. A Web-supported course may or may not *require* students to use the Internet. For those who have no personal access, the instructor may provide the materials through class, library, or lab. The university may provide access through student computer labs or in student dormitories. Access to the course Internet site may be open or password-protected. Typically, a Web-supported course will offer an on-line discussion board or chat room to enhance class discussions. In addition to traditional student-faculty interactions, a Web-supported course usually makes a faculty E-mail address available to students for additional interaction opportunities. Students also may have special group "meetings" via computer conferencing technology. Both real-time and virtual meetings can be supported in the Internet environment. Also, students can obtain more information about course topics through either personal or faculty-guided Web searches. The two key criteria for a Web-supported course are that (1) an on-campus classroom component is required, and (2) at least some of the course materials are available on the Web (although the course may permit students to obtain all their materials without accessing the Web).

A *Web-based course* is one in which the entire course is on-line. This modality requires that all students have access to the Internet. The syllabus, including course description, objectives, class schedule (if any), handouts, examinations, class discussions, and so on are all available only through the Internet. Texts and other required materials that must be purchased are available by mail from the university bookstore. Students typically communicate with each other and the faculty via a discussion board, chat room, and/or E-mail. Faculty may or may not provide lecture materials to support required readings. Typically, faculty provide information about important links to relevant sites on the Web, but students are also expected to do considerable work in personal searches to enhance their own learning.[1] A Web-based course may or may not adhere to the traditional semester or quarter schedule of the university in which it is housed. Web courses, like correspondence courses, may permit the student wide latitude about scheduling readings, homework, projects, and examinations. The three key criteria for a Web-based course are as follows:

1. There is no on-campus requirement for any part of the course. This means that everything, from registration, enrollment, and payment of tuition and fees to content presentations and group projects, can be handled through the Internet. Thus, students who live in the same city as the university have no advantage over students who live halfway around the world.
2. All of the required course materials are either available on-line or may be purchased from the university bookstore or other mail-order supplier.
3. Students who live at a great distance from each other and from the faculty can communicate with faculty and other students via E-mail and perhaps through some combination of discussion boards, computer conferencing, or chat rooms, although phone calls may be used occasionally.

ADVANTAGES AND LIMITATIONS OF THESE EDUCATIONAL MODALITIES

Traditional On-Campus Courses

Traditional on-campus courses offer many advantages. The format is familiar to students who have attended high school. The daily or weekly class schedule and deadlines for papers, projects, and exams provide a form of external discipline. The instructor and student have the advantage of face-to-face discussions. This is perhaps the greatest advantage the traditional classroom format can offer. Students and faculty mutually benefit from vigorous intellectual discussions about the content of the course. When students and faculty discuss problems, identify potential solutions, and hear each other's ideas, a great deal of learning can take place. All can hear the words, inflections, and feeling tone of each other's utterances and at the same time gain further information from body language—both of the speaker and of the listeners. Of course, the teacher ensures that content is current and can offer personal support to the student who struggles with some of the content. This modality has been in use for as long as formal education has existed because it is so successful for most people.

This format does create some problems. First, the student must arrange his or her schedule to fit the scheduled time of the course. This requirement may exclude many people from the class, simply due to scheduling problems. Second, for many students, travel to and from the university and parking are significant problems. For many graduate students, class attendance requires a 2- or 3-hour drive. Our classes meet only once a week for 3 hours; but adding in the drive, students must allocate 7 to 9 hours per week just for class attendance. Homework, study, and library time require another 9 hours. Parking at our university is a problem. Most universities were built for the use of young (17–22-year-old) students who lived on campus in dormitories or one or two blocks away in student housing. These students walk to classes, libraries, and university activities. None of our graduate students and fewer than half of our undergraduate students fit this profile. For some people, physical disabilities are such that attendance at a traditional classroom course is not possible. Third, although this format allows for in-class discussion, those discussions must be very limited in time. Classrooms are often in demand, and the students and instructor must vacate in time for the next class to begin. Fourth, shy students are at a great disadvantage. Particularly in large classes, only brave or aggressive students may get the chance to ask their questions or offer their opinions. In fact, in classes with more than 12–15 students, somebody will almost always be overlooked.

Correspondence Courses

Correspondence courses have long offered an educational opportunity to people whose location or job made traditional classroom education impossible. They have also been an important resource to people whose physical disabilities make it impossible to attend a regular classroom. Many people living in areas far from colleges and universities do not have the money to give up work and move to a college location. Some people are employed in jobs that require a great deal of travel; others are required to work rotating shifts; still others live too far from a college or for other reasons are unable to meet the requirements of a traditional classroom schedule. In the past, correspondence courses offered one of the few options for college credit to all these people. Most correspondence courses provide generous deadlines for course completion. For people who learn in ways different from those of typical students and who therefore cannot succeed in a traditional classroom, correspondence courses may facilitate learning success by allowing the student to take all the time needed to learn and may give students more latitude to use personally developed learning techniques.

The correspondence course format does have some drawbacks. First, by its nature, it offers limited faculty support. This is a barrier to students when their reading materials are insufficient or when the student's work processes are ineffective. Second, for many students, the student-to-student interaction can facilitate great learning. Unfortunately, there is little to no student cohort support available in a correspondence course format. Third, correspondence courses may not work well for highly changeable content. The materials must be prepared months or even years in advance, and updates may be difficult to incorporate into the course. For some types of courses, such as computing, advertising, and medical topics, changes in the field may occur so rapidly that the correspondence course format simply cannot keep up. Fourth, correspondence courses have a much higher noncompletion rate than the other formats presented in this chapter. This is probably a function of all of the above factors. It may also be due to the lack of human contact. The need to communicate with a teacher on a regular basis can serve as a strong impetus to study and prepare so as to avoid losing face.

Web-supported Courses

Web-supported courses are essentially enhanced traditional courses. They have generally the same advantages and disadvantages as traditional courses have. The Web is used as an additional learning opportunity and may greatly increase communication among faculty and students. It also may ease some of the problems of obtaining syllabi, class handouts, and other paper materials because copying expenses are increasingly restricted by most universities. It is also cheaper for the student to download these materials than to have to purchase them from the campus bookstore or copying center. Web-support courses may greatly enhance the value of the course to shy students who are unlikely to speak up in class. If the Web supports include E-mail to faculty and other students or chat room or discussion board facilities, the student's shyness may cease to be a problem. Shyness is generally a reticence in the physical presence of others. However, most shy people feel quite comfortable with computer communications.

Web-based Courses

This relatively new modality offers nothing essentially new to the educational process but, properly handled, may combine advantages of several of the other modalities. As with traditional on-campus courses, personal communications among teachers and students are a great strength of the format. Although contact is remote, it can (and should) be frequent. The best Internet teachers plan to answer E-mail from students daily or at least two to three times per week. Students often form on-line study and project groups, and those students will often communicate with each other several times a day. The students may lose some communicative power because of the loss of physical/visual contact during communication. However, that may not be much of a factor as students become more accustomed to the Internet.

Even though people are not physically together at all and may not even be together simultaneously, they are still able to communicate effectively if they have any degree of comfort with computers. More and more people have grown accustomed to personal and business use of E-mail, chat rooms, and discussion boards. Many believe they are able to communicate *better* through the computer than in person. They believe there is less miscommunication because the written word can be viewed and edited prior to sending it, and inadvertent negative voice tones do not occur. One is less likely to blurt out something untoward when the communication is written. Also, nobody is ever interrupted.

One great advantage of Web courses is their effect on people who have physical (speech or hearing) disabilities or who are just quiet or shy by nature. None of these characteristics has anything to do with intelligence, creativity, or potential class contributions. However, these kinds of barriers can seriously interfere with a student's ability to participate as a full member of the class. Unfortunately, human prejudice being what it is, class members also may misinterpret another's disability as a lack of intelligence. Essentially, the Web wipes out the effects of all of these problems.

As previously mentioned, shyness and most physical disabilities are not factors in writing or computer communications. People who are typically quiet in a group often find lots to communicate via the computer. Shyness (and quietness may be a form of shyness) is typically a reaction to the physical presence in one location of many strangers or casual acquaintances. Students in our Internet classes have often told us they have never before felt so comfortable participating fully in a class. They are amazed and delighted that shyness is simply not a factor in Internet courses. As teachers, we find this a truly delightful effect. The input of people with a history of withholding their comments in class because of disabilities of one kind or another often proves to be astute, interesting, and highly stimulating to the entire class.

Other advantages include the ability of students to do classwork at their own convenience. Students who travel can take along a portable computer. As long as their Internet service provider (ISP) is a national service with local phone numbers in most areas, students can do classwork anywhere and anytime. The student may have to travel to a location where there is no local phone number for the ISP. Good organization can work to keep long-distance calls to the ISP very short. The student can call in and download lectures and discussion items to the hard drive and then sign off the Internet. The student can then study the materials on the laptop computer. Students should always use a word processor to construct their papers. E-mail items and discussion board items also can be constructed locally. Then, with a short second long-distance call to the ISP, the student simply uses the "cut and paste" facilities to move communications from local programs to the course Internet site. Costly calls might be occasioned only if a student wishes to do a lengthy search on the Internet for further information on a class topic. However, many students will organize their time in such a way that those searches are scheduled when they have access to a local number for their ISP.

The final advantage of Web-based courses is that they satisfy customer demand. More and more people are asking that courses and whole degree programs be offered on-line. The convenience is becoming increasingly critical to adult students. Student demand for on-line courses may force colleges and universities to choose between offering more and more of their courses on-line or downsizing to fit the reduced number of traditional on-campus students.

Web-based courses do have some disadvantages. First, the student must have access to a computer and an Internet link. Not everybody has this technology in the home or office. If students have to come to campus anyway to use computer labs, several of the key advantages of an on-line course are lost. Second, some students are simply not computer-literate; for them this modality may be ineffective. However, this disadvantage should decline over time. During the next 10 years more and more college students will have grown up using computers and the Internet in school and in their personal lives. They will feel as comfortable with Internet communications as they do with physical-presence communication.

Third, although the Internet is quite adaptable to most theory courses, there remain many challenges to teaching hands-on content through this medium. Even more important is the need to personally watch students perform tasks if their skill level is to be assessed. For example, there have been many films developed for medical and nursing students on how to start an intravenous (IV) infusion. However, watching a film will never produce a competent practitioner. The students typically practice on an artificial arm model and perhaps on teachers and other students before attempting to start an IV on a patient. Much development on how to use the Internet to teach and evaluate skill tasks remains to be done before certain kinds of courses can be offered on-line. One way this problem can be addressed is to reduce rather than eliminate on-campus course work. Some programs require students to come on-campus for a period of time, such as a summer, for some of their work. Then the bulk of their content courses are provided on-line.

Fourth, most teachers are not yet sufficiently familiar with the Internet and with this format as an educational tool to function as instructors of Internet courses. Many are highly resistant to learning. And in fact, access to education on Internet teaching is limited. These problems will probably be solved over time, but in the early 2000s they will be significant barriers to the development of on-line course offerings.

Fifth, there may be some loss of learning due to the loss of face-to-face class discussions. Personally, we do not give this argument much credence. The evidence to date shows that learning for Internet courses equals and sometimes even exceeds learning in the traditional classroom format. However, the political fallout from the argument about the credibility of on-line courses is a great disadvantage at this time. Many members of university faculties are extremely skeptical of using the Internet to offer courses. They refuse to prepare their courses for the on-line format and politick against their departments' and universities' moving in this direction. We suspect much of this resistance is occasioned more by personal fear of having to change their teaching approach than by honest consideration of evidence of poor learning in Internet courses. The many concerns about lower learning for students in on-line courses have not been validated, and personal experience has shown these authors that learning levels in both modalities are highly dependent upon student commitment to learning. In fact, some people who are very popular classroom teachers may not be able to adapt to the new format. Some experts can, with very little preparation time, simply enter the classroom and give a fine lecture. This approach is not appropriate for the Internet. Thus, for at least some faculty, Internet courses will require much more work than traditional classroom courses.

Sixth, this modality is so new that the infrastructure to support Web-based courses may be inadequate in many colleges. Teachers may have to spend a great deal of time at the beginning of the semester helping their students get registered with the university and enrolled in the course, obtaining course passwords, and making sure that the students are able to work with the technology used in the course. In a traditional course the registrar's office, the bookstore, and lab assistants handle these kinds of things. Typically, faculty are not paid more for this extra work and are not given higher credit for teaching an on-line course. Thus, this work may not be counted in the teacher's workload. That, of course, means that the teacher donates all that work. This is a disadvantage because it will increase teacher resistance to the modality.

Seventh, issues of copyright, privacy, security, plagiarism, and authentication of student work constitute special problems for Internet courses. On-campus courses have library reserve desks where a teacher can place a copy of a journal article, book, or other material that he or she wishes to share with students. Copyright laws forbid the teacher, bookstore, and copy center to make copies for all the students unless permission is obtained, and usually, a royalty is paid to the copyright owner. Of course, in the library, each student can make a personal copy, so the effect is the same as the teacher or bookstore making copies. In a Web-based course this approach doesn't work. The teacher or university must make contact with the owner of the copyright and either buy reprints or pay a royalty for making copies. The students buy the reprints with their course packet (that includes texts and other materials purchased through the bookstore).

Faculty always have to be concerned that students may submit purchased term papers and other students' work as their own. There are public sites on the Web that sell papers for this very purpose. This is a serious problem in America. One of the reasons our educational system is so well respected and that our students are marketable all over the world is the rigor of our coursework. If students begin to pass with high grades without doing the necessary work to earn the grade, a college degree from an American university will soon become less valuable. All parts of the system must guard against cheating and grade inflation. Employers hire graduates with the understanding that the college degree is backed by a considerable knowledge base and certain writing, critical thinking, and analytic skills. Unfortunately, Web courses do not offer any better protections against dishonesty than do classroom courses. In fact, for exams, the Web-based courses do have one disadvantage: closed-book exams are much more difficult to achieve. Also, it can be difficult to prevent several students from getting together and taking the exams together. In a traditional classroom the teacher knows who the students are; in very large exam rooms, sometimes students must present their picture ID, which is checked against the class list.

There are some ways to help ensure an honest exam. In the past we have had students identify a teacher, department chair, or other school official in a community college or university near the student's home to proctor the exam. The student had to contract with the proctor and provide us with the proctor's name, title, address, and phone number 30 days in advance of the exam. We verified the identity of the proctor by calling the school and checking on his or her employment position and then calling the proctor to discuss a mutually agreeable exam process. We then faxed the exam to the proctor the day prior to the exam, and the proctor faxed the completed exam back to me immediately after the exam was completed. There are companies such as the American College Testing Corporation (ACT) that will provide a computer and proctor for exams for a fee. Of course, these preparations are extra work, but these examples show that there are ways to accomplish proctored examinations for Web-based courses.

Another method that has worked well is the use of integrative essay exams. We develop exam questions that require the student to integrate and analyze course information. They are open-book, open-notes exams, and we allow several days for completion. Several of our students have commented that the exams took 6–8 hours to complete. However, they also said that they learned a huge amount from the exams because the questions helped them think through the meaning of the content in the text and class notes.

COMMON MYTHS OF WEB-BASED COURSES

Faculty Can Accommodate More Students by Using Technology

This myth is particularly damaging to a school's efforts to get a program started. It frightens teachers because they actually need *small* classes to start with. A Web-based course may increase the size of those classes that tend to have a small local enrollment. The distance opportunity increased our Informatics course from 7 to 25 the year after we began offering it on-line. The point is that the Web format will help fill classes. It does not reduce faculty workload for a given course.

Using Technology Saves the Institution Money

Ultimately, this may not be fiction, but today it is just not generally true. Money can be saved if one teacher can handle a much larger number of students. However, programs that are successful will not generally have extremely large student-to-faculty ratios. If the students cannot get timely responses to their questions, they will find another school that provides sufficient faculty time. Some schools hope to make money by attracting more out-of-state students, who pay much higher tuition. Only time will prove this true or false. In the late 1990s many schools had to offer in-state tuition to Internet students to fill classes. Over time, we suspect that prestigious schools that offer a full degree program will be able to fill Internet classes, even at out-of-state tuition costs. Schools that offer only isolated courses or whose reputation is not world-class will have to offer cheaper tuition to fill classes. Money also can be saved if the number of buildings (and attendant maintenance costs) can be reduced. Internet students do not use the classrooms or student activity buildings that traditional campuses must provide. We suspect that eventually, if enough students opt for on-line courses, the number and size of buildings can be reduced.

Technology saves the faculty member time. Similar to the previous myth, this ultimately may prove true. However, it is not true today. The development time needed for a Web-based course is much greater than that for a traditional course. Faculty workload must be greatly reduced when a teacher is first learning to teach on-line. The first time we taught a course on-line, we spent approximately 30 hours per week on that one course. We were learning to use the technology, developing and trying out new ways to offer material, and experiencing the inefficiency of any beginner. Today, we can teach that same course much more efficiently and spend about the same amount of time on that course as we do for on-campus courses. Of course, since we can do that course at our convenience rather than on the university's class schedule, it sometimes seems easier to teach that course than to teach on-campus courses. Once the lectures are developed, the faculty will still need to review and update them every semester, just as they do with on-campus courses.

"If I can't see the students, I cannot teach the class effectively." *Au contraire!* We get to know many of our Internet students much better than many of my on-campus students. We may or may not have a picture of the student, but we certainly communicate personally with most students at least once per week. Human personalities come through computer communications quite nicely. Sometimes we think we get to know our Internet students even better. There is a feeling of equality about the Web that many students don't experience in person. Our Web students are free to address us by our first names; they often share their personal as well as professional and learning joys and problems with us, and we continue to hear from many of them today, even though they completed our course years ago. That long-term relationship does not always happen, but it adds greatly to the joy of teaching as a career choice. We certainly develop as great a feeling of fondness for our Internet students as we do for our on-campus students. The one thing we miss about Internet students is that we do not get to hug each other when they submit an outstanding piece of work, or just generally want to express their affection.

KEY ISSUES IN DELIVERING CONTENT TO DISTANCE STUDENTS

Key issues involved in using the Internet to deliver distance courses include (1) knowing your customer, (2) development of a student facilitation model of teaching, (3) preservation of academic standards, and (4) registration and enrollment issues. There is much to think through in each of these areas if a high-quality, credible educational program is to be offered through the Internet.

Who Is the Customer?

In this media, more than in any other, students are your customers. Clearly, each student must be must be given a good education and should receive good service from the entire educational institution, from the registrar and teacher to the support staff. As more colleges and universities get into the business of offering on-line courses, students have more choices. Thus, it is important to market to potential students, and part of marketing is excellent service. The student should be able to discover your on-line program through trade journals, Internet search engines, and professional contacts. Every university should have an on-line registration and enroll-ment system. Students should not have to use the U.S. postal service (called "snail mail" by E-mail users). One of the problems for graduate students is the need to contact their undergraduate universities by mail to get transcripts. It is important that universities develop a system whereby a student can pay for a transcript on-line with a credit card, and the university simply E-mails the transcript to the graduate school or department where the student plans to enroll. In our experience, this transcript issue has caused too many delays in enrollment.

Students are your most immediate customers. They are neither your only nor your most important customer. The most important customer is the future employer of your graduates. It is important for *all* faculty to maintain a relationship with community employers, and if possible, with the national employer community. We regularly meet with local directors of nursing and agency CEOs to talk about what they think we should include in our courses. We have department meetings with these people to consult with them on the full curriculum. Maintaining close contact with the world in which your students are expected to function is essential to the quality of your content.

Ultimately, your customer is all of society. In publicly owned schools, taxes provide at least some of the support for overhead, faculty salaries, and other costs. Even if none of the costs are tax-supported, the value of your educational offerings will ultimately be judged by society's respect for your graduates. It is important to maintain the goodwill of the public because schools are social institutions. If your graduates have poor skills, ultimately your reputation will suffer; and parents, teachers, high school counselors, and other advisors will not encourage students to seek their education from your school. Both faculty and students are ultimately public relations representatives for your school. It is everybody's job to ensure that a degree from your institution is treated with respect and admiration everywhere.

Maintain Extremely High Academic Standards

Students must leave your course with marketable new knowledge and skills. If the degree your university confers is not backed by solid knowledge and skills, the value of a degree from your institution will decline. We once knew of a vice president of nursing who would not hire nursing graduates with master's degrees from the local university. She claimed that their degrees were given too easily and that the students could not communicate well in writing. She further noted that if their skills were not significantly improved over the skills of the other nurses, she could find no justification for paying them more. In another case, where there was much cheating in a computer programming department, the university began having trouble placing students in local businesses. Students found they had to leave town to find a job because employers had no faith in their work skills and work habits.

University Faculty Evaluation Committees

Such groups must be extremely careful with interpretation of student evaluations of faculty and courses. In our opinion, the student's evaluation should be linked with the student's course grade. If it can be demonstrated that evaluations correlate highly with student grades, then only the A students' course evaluations should be considered in faculty evaluations. Faculty members are smart, and if they find that their job evaluations and merit raises are dependent on making every student happy with them, grade inflation is the only possible result. Ultimately, grade inflation is the fault of the system, not of the individual teacher. This is true of all courses, but especially of on-line courses because of the great personal discipline required of distance students.

Use Every Technique You Can Find to Make Learning Easy

Make difficult content as easy to learn as possible by reducing the red tape and unnecessary bureaucracy as much as possible, not by "dumbing down" your content and expectations. Be meticulous about organizing the material in such a way that learning proceeds logically. Avoid jumping back and forth among topics. Make the course and module objectives explicit, clear, and measurable. For example, avoid objectives such as "The student will understand how to start an IV." A better objective might be "The student will list the five principles of starting an IV and will successfully demonstrate the technique." Course and module objectives must be behavioral, measurable, and clearly linked to both individual class session objectives and to assignments, projects, and examinations.

Make Sure That Screens on the Web-based Course Have Good Eye Appeal

Colors used should provide good contrast so that the student can read text. Never use pastel text on a light background. Use large print and easy-to-read print fonts, such as Arial or Times Roman, so that students don't get eyestrain. Color, font style and size, and movement (such as that found in animation) can be used to draw attention to important points and maintain interest. Present content in the same order as you listed the objectives to make it easy for students to follow the learning trajectory you planned for your course.

Make Learning Fun

Develop or search out public domain case studies that make learning difficult content fun. A teacher should strive to be an entertainer as well as a conveyer of knowledge. Remember the history of the television show *All in the Family*. It used comedy, lovable and sometimes unlovable characters, and drama to make some very important points about human dignity and justice. Even people who were reared in racist environments watched that show despite the fact that its content was diametrically opposed to their personal beliefs. It probably brought home the unfairness and wrongness of racial and ethnic discrimination to many people who would otherwise never have questioned their beliefs.

People learn and retain knowledge better when it is fun to learn. We have had games in our courses in which the students had a contest to find the best sites for things like ergonomics research. We also had a game in which students were asked to find one credible and one untrustworthy site for a particular medical problem. They had to search out the Internet and the professional literature to find out who the author was, if the author had a professional affiliation with a credible institution, and if he or she was providing professional information or personal opinion. Several students have since told us that ever since that game they never again assumed that something on the Web was valid; they always check out the source. Some things will always require hard study and work. (Children still have to memorize the multiplication tables.) But teachers should always remember that learning is much easier and better retained when teachers and parents can make a game of learning.

Make Sure That Every Part of the Course Contributes to Achieving the Stated Course Objectives

Ensure that class "lectures," case studies, and assignments are designed to assist the student to achieve the stated objectives. Students legitimately dislike busywork. They resent assignments if they cannot understand why they are doing it. Good teachers give assignments that are designed to meet explicit learning objectives, and the learning materials should make clear what each part of the course contributes to the students' learning process.

Real-Time Requirements

Decide whether or not to require any real-time learning experiences. Chat rooms and audioconferencing technology can be an effective way to provide for class discussion and can give teachers an important outlet for their need to personally share their expertise with students in a direct way. However, real-time experiences may be inconvenient in the extreme for students who live in widely different time zones. If the student body is limited to North and South America, a reasonable time for a real-time experience might be noon Central Standard Time (CST). That would have students in the east on line at 1:00 p.m., Mountain Standard Time students would get on-line at 11:00 a.m., Pacific Standard Time students would join the class at 10:00 a.m., Alaska at 9:00 a.m., the Aleutian islands at 8:00 a.m. Students in Hawaii would have to sign on at 7:00 a.m. A real-time experience scheduled for 8:00 a.m. Eastern Standard Time requires Californians to sign on at 5:00 a.m. and Hawaiians at 2:00 a.m. Clearly, the course that has students from around the world must carefully consider any real-time experiences.

Develop Assignments and Explicit Grading Criteria

Make assignments and grading criteria available to students in the syllabus. An advantage of Internet courses is that they can allow students the ability to plan their own classwork schedules and to do the work at their own pace and convenience. Distance students often are people with erratic and demanding work schedules who work in nontraditional ways. For example, a student may have no time to work on the course one week but may spend two or three entire days another week. Instructors also must control their schedules. Therefore, the fact that a student submits an assignment early does not necessarily mean that the faculty has to grade it early. Students like quick feedback, so the syllabus should clearly state that early papers may not be graded until the due date because due dates are one way teachers plan their own work schedules.

Do have due dates. Due dates help students discipline themselves to get projects done. The teacher should give consideration to having grade penalties for late work. However, working adults will sometimes need extensions. We find it most helpful to require students to ask for extensions and always include a new due date for the extension. Procrastinators may be poorly disciplined, but they may also be people who have great need for flexibility because of work and family demands. The most successful attitude is directed toward facilitating students' work, not toward punitive actions. We contract, cajole, and encourage students to get their work in. We are not comfortable threatening students with an F grade except in the most extreme cases. For example, we must remind students of the consequence of noncompletion when they still haven't completed their work more than a month or two after the end of the course. Some students do find after they enroll that they simply do not have what it takes to complete an on-line course. Despite our flexibility, it is always students' responsibility to manage their time.

Withdrawal dates should be generous. People should have at least until midterm to withdraw without receiving an F. The teacher should schedule enough assignments during the first half of the course so that the heaviest workload hits in the first 4 weeks. That way, students will have a chance to determine early if they can't handle the workload. To repeat, it is best for the teacher to view the relationship as facilitative, not punitive.

Take an Active Role in Facilitating Class Discussion

Most students will not use the discussion facilities unless it is a class requirement. They begin by greatly preferring to communicate only with the instructor via E-mail. This practice *must* be discouraged! Students need to use each other as resources, and teachers must protect their own time. It is not efficient to answer the same question 25 times to individuals. We always copy student content questions onto the discussion board and respond to them there. Soon, students learn to use the board for content questions.

The best technique we have found is to have a discussion board assignment the very first week. This approach also helps my Internet support personnel manage their time. We simply let them know that the first week or two students will be required to use the discussion board, so that is when most of those technical questions will arise. Some students will have to be nudged occasionally with an E-mail suggesting that they make some entries on the board. In most classes, there will be some eager users and some who just don't care to participate much in the class discussion. However, we have had people who were very quiet in an on-campus course who became the busiest users of the discussion board. Shyness isn't the barrier here. Students' time pressures may be a factor.

HINTS ON GOOD WEB COURSE DESIGN

- Do not get too fancy. A good design is a simple one. Limit the use of frames technology unless it is central to the navigation scheme.
- Legibility is extremely important. Do not make the user squint to read your text. Large, sans serif fonts (such as Arial) work best.
- Provide users the guide to where they are in relation to the entire page. This can be accomplished with visual indicators, page numbers, and a variety of other techniques.
- Be consistent. Provide users with the same navigation features in predictable locations on the screen. Do not get fancy or be moving things around. Decide on a template and stick with it.
- Provide basic information about the course and instructor. For instance, an instructor bio with information on how to contact you is critical. Use the school or company logo on the opening page. Identify the course and provide an area for visitors to E-mail for further information.
- Create an index page that provides users with an easy way to get to specific information.
- Provide users with links to support services, embedded into your course; for instance, links to the library, bookstore, registrar's office, financial aid, and the like.
- Avoid embedding fancy things, like Java-based applets (calculators, etc.) unless you are sure the students have a browser that is Java-enabled.
- Make the course multisensory, multidimensional. Do not limit the course to a "computer textbook" but instead consider using the power of the Internet to enhance the course with audio, video, photos, animation, interactive testing, and so on.

- Develop an evaluation/feedback instrument for the course. Encourage feedback following every unit or module.
- The course home page is a marketing tool. Obtain professional consultation and design services to be sure it is very attractive and interesting. Of course, if must be easy to find.

MARKET YOUR COURSE

- Faculty responsible for the course should ensure that an attractive, informative course home page is created and maintained as a marketing tool.
- Register the course with as many search engines as possible.
- Register the course with *The World Lecture Hall*.
- Be sure that program fliers and other promotional materials include the course home page address as well as a course listing and course description.
- Try to get a paper or news article about your course published in local, regional, and national professional newspapers or journals.
- Advertise your Web-based educational offerings in magazines and journals targeted at your potential student audience.
- Be sure that your university, college, and department home pages have prominent links to your course.
- Be sure that your course home page has links to the school's admissions and enrollment Web pages.
- Your home page should have a clearly marked link to on-line course registration (if it exists) or to an E-mail address where potential students can request enrollment forms.

NOTES

1. A rule of thumb for graduate school is as follows:
   For every credit hour, allow 3 hours of work outside class for homework, reading, library time, and student projects. Therefore, a three-credit course should take the student 12 hours per week—3 hours of class time and 9 hours outside class. The rule for undergraduate courses is generally 2 hours of work for every credit hour plus in-class time. These are only general rules; students who have difficulty with the material may need more time, and students with a special aptitude or prior training may need less time.

3

Software Tools for Web Course Development

Robert Gibson and Mary L. McHugh

When developing either an entirely on-line–delivered course or a Web-enhanced traditional course, there are a variety of sophisticated software applications designed to facilitate the development process. These applications are available for instructors in the K–12 environment, higher education, or even corporate training scenarios. Typically, the institution or organization settles on a software application that will complement the mission of the institution and that can be adequately supported by the technical personnel. To complicate matters, however, new course development technologies emerge on a frequent basis that add tempting new enhancements and features. To understand the differences we will briefly visit some of the various types of applications currently available for Web course development.

ON-LINE LEARNING ENVIRONMENTS

Although sometimes referred to as *course support systems*, this category of application software is specifically designed for Internet course delivery. These programs are commonly considered turnkey applications because they provide a reasonably simple, step-by-step approach to developing either a Web-based or Web-enhanced course. That is to say, they are generally designed around a template architecture that is divided into various categories, such as peer-to-peer or student-instructor collaboration, assessment, course management, and course didactics. Instructors are not required to have any technical understanding of the programming, coding, or Web server processes. Rather, the instructor simply completes the course information following the requisite steps provided within the application. The majority of these applications are driven through a Web interface. That is, the instructor need simply have access to a networked Web browser to access and design the content. The course developer can add, delete, or update information from an office, home, or even hotel room. These programs allow various files to be uploaded and hosted, such as PowerPoint or Excel files. Popular applications of this type include Web Course-in-a-Box, developed in association with Virginia Commonwealth; WebCT (www.webct.com), developed in association with the University of British Columbia; TopClass (www.topclass.com), developed by a corporation in Dublin, Ireland; Courseinfo (www.blackboard.com), developed in association with Cornell University; and LearningSpace (www.learningspace.com), developed by IBM.

On-line learning environments are currently being used by hundreds of colleges and universities. According to Robson (1999), there are presently between 50 and 100 individual products that qualify as course-support systems. Each of these applications has undergone a series of upgrades and enhancements over the past years that provide an increasingly vast array of very sophisticated course components. The most sophisticated of these applications even provides the ability to connect directly to campus registration systems, such as PeopleSoft, to import course roster information. Generally, however, these applications provide a similar set of components:

1. *Course communication features*, including a discussion board, chat client, and E-mail; collaborative whiteboard.
2. *Course assessment features* that provide a variety of multiple choice, T/F, matching, and short-answer assessments that can be delivered at predetermined times. Tests can be randomized and delivered via test banks.
3. *Course management features*, that include an on-line grade book, course rosters, student access tracking, and student password information.
4. *Course information features*, including a syllabus, instructor home page, calendar, and course announcements.

5. *Course didactic features*, including file uploading capabilities (PowerPoint, Word, and other related course files), streaming video and audio files, external Web links, drill-and-practice and simulation exercises, and course module builders.

These types of applications provide several advantages for an instructor. First, they allow the instructor to retain control of the course. Instructors are often at the mercy of a support unit to update course materials on a timely basis. Often, these support units are overwhelmed with requests for Web updates and changes. Using this type of application, the instructor need simply log into his or her course through a Web browser (from work, home, or wherever they happen to have access to a networked computer) to update content. As soon as the instructor saves the changes, the Web page is automatically updated for the students. No special transferring of material is required between a workstation and a server.

Second, these applications are often very easy to use. These programs are designed to facilitate the course creation process with little technical overhead. However, certain on-line learning environment applications are designed with better user interface considerations than others have, making these applications easier to utilize. Additionally, these applications remove much of the need for special interface and graphic design skills, which, if lacking, can actually *impede* the effectiveness of a Web-delivered course.

Perhaps the biggest disadvantage can also be considered yet another asset: the nature of these programs means that courses themselves often look very similar. There is often not a tremendous amount of flexibility provided in these programs for personalizing the look and feel, with the exception of colors and perhaps a few graphic elements. This lack of flexibility is enough to dissuade some instructors from employing this type of program. However, the continuity of the program does provide students with a familiar interface, assuming several instructors are utilizing the same application. Consistent features that are in familiar screen locations reduce student confusion.

Third, there has been some criticism regarding the lack of standards for these applications. The criticism was directed at the companies for not implementing an easy means to transport courses developed on one platform to a competing platform used at another institution, in the event that the instructor moved. This standards issue is being addressed through a consortium referred to as the EDUCAUSE IMS (Instructional Management System) Project that is encouraging the various companies to implement a standards-based system to ease in the portability of courses designed using the various products (www.imsproject.org).

WEB PAGE DEVELOPMENT APPLICATIONS

This category of software includes those programs that are not expressly designed for Web *course* development but rather Web *page* development in general. Perhaps the best metaphor for describing this category of Web page development applications is simply a blank canvas. Using this type of program, the instructor can design the course in nearly unlimited styles, depending on his or her imagination and creativity. Many instructors choose to use this type of application for this very reason. The on-line learning environment applications approximate a "paint-by-numbers" because the basic course template is already in place. Using the latter, an instructor need simply populate the information in the predetermined categories and fields. This is not the case with Web page development applications. Essentially, the instructor or course designer must create the various categories and links manually. In addition, the graphic elements must be created by using third-party applications uploaded to a server. This can be time-consuming; however, it does provide nearly unlimited flexibility.

Popular applications of this type include Microsoft FrontPage (www.microsoft.com), Macromedia DreamWeaver (www.macromedia. com), and Adobe PageMill (www.adobe.com). These programs typically require the purchase of a client application that can be legally installed on both an office computer and a home computer. To achieve full functionality, a network administrator establishes an account on a Web server that can provide for additional features and extensibility, often referred to as *server extensions*. The advantage these programs have lies in the file management system and design features. FrontPage, for instance, employs a sophisticated file management component that closely echoes the Windows Explorer. Directories and files can be created, deleted, and renamed with relative ease. Additionally, changes to a link in one page will cascade throughout the site to change other pages that might also be affected, freeing the designer from having to manually edit links. FrontPage 2000 boasts an even richer set of management features, allowing a designer to publisher other Microsoft Office applications to the Web with relative ease.

Like FrontPage, DreamWeaver employs a sophisticated array of course design features, such as animated effects, forms processing, and a variety of enhanced graphic elements. The instructor or course developer can either design in a graphic environment or, if comfortable with scripting languages, may switch to the scripting view to develop the content by using code. Either way, these programs are extremely powerful for any type of Web application.

The primary disadvantage these programs have, versus the on-line learning environments, is that they often do not incorporate the rich tool set of course-specific features. For example, they do not have a native assessment engine, grade book, or communications program. At the same time, using special features available within these programs, a creative instructor or course developer could customize these components from scratch, assuming the instructor possesses programming skills.

COMMUNICATIONS

Communications in a course can be handled in a number of ways. Typically, on-line courses employ E-mail, chat, a discussion board, and/or a list serve. Here is the difference: E-mail, of course, is the basic communications vehicle provided in any on-line course. It must be available to facilitate communication between students and between instructor and students.

Chat, on the other hand, is a *synchronous* communications system, engaging the learners in on-line communication *at the same time*. Using chat, students type comments and questions into a field that resembles E-mail. However, the communication is instantaneous, so the response is delivered to other participants immediately. Chat is fast and furious and requires a short, abbreviated writing style. Chat clients are generally free. There are many available on the Internet, including the popular mIRC. However, finding a private room in which to conduct class can be challenging. Your institution will have to establish chat services on a local server in order to ensure privacy.

A discussion board, on the other hand, is perhaps one of the most popular communications systems for on-line learning. Using a discussion board, the course dialogue is logged in a hierarchical format referred to as "threads." Students may review the threads at any time and add comments or questions at their leisure. This type of communications system is akin to E-mail in that it is *asynchronous*, or *not at the same time*. However, the advantage of a discussion board lies in the hierarchical threads that can viewed at any time and archived following the completion of the course. Popular discussion boards include Allaire Forums (www. allaire.com) and WebBoard. WebBoard (www.webboard.com) even includes a chat component.

Finally, list serves, or discussion lists, allow participants to communicate via a private forum. Joining a list allows any communications to be pushed automatically to each subscriber via the E-mail system. Think of it as course communication that is automatically delivered to your inbox. The advantage of this system is convenience. Users do not have to open a special program, other than their E-mail, to read the course content. However, the messages are not organized in any logical fashion, and they generally are not archived. This can lead to disjointed communications between participants. For instance, if a student posts a response to a question using a list serve but does not reference the question properly, every participant may see a message come through with something short and confusing like "Yes. I agree. But what do you think?" A popular list serve application is Major Domo. It must be installed on a server at your location; however, the cost is generally reasonable or even free.

ASSESSMENT APPLICATIONS

A variety of assessment applications are available for course designers. Most of the on-line learning environment applications feature a sophisticated course assessment engine. However, there are many freestanding assessment applications that provide a rich tool set for developing on-line tests. The problem with on-line testing is validity and verification: who is actually out there taking the test? A variety of technologies have been proposed that could assist an instructor with verification, such as retinal scanning and fingerprint analysis. However, even the best technologies cannot prevent cheating. Unfortunately, there is no easy answer to the question of on-line testing verification. Many instructors who favor on-line testing are quick to point out that courses offered in large lecture halls have no more security than an on-line test, but this explanation does not satisfy the pundits. Regardless, these testing applications are generally quite sophisticated and add a tempting array of options. Most offer multiple choice (with distracter unlimited options), true/false, matching, short answer, fill-in-the-blank, and survey-type questions. Many have the ability to include graphics in the question set and can provide "one-at-a-time" test questioning. Researchers who are interested in collecting data can use these applications to survey participants, freeing them from sending out costly paper-based surveys.

In addition to featuring a wide variety of test types, these quizzing programs often have the ability to generate random test sets from a large bank of questions. Course designers also can set the tests to be available for a predetermined period or be available only for a certain time following the start of the test by a student (timed tests). To access the test, students must input a password supplied by the course designer or instructor. Tests can be set for drill and practice or for keeps. Tests also can be set to provide feedback to the student if the instructor intends the test to be a tutorial.

QuestionMark's Perception (www.questionmark.com) is one such assessment application that provides a rich variety of testing tools. Using Perception, results can be collected in a database and later exported to a spreadsheet or statistical program for analysis. MoneyTree's QuizPlease (www.quizplease.com) provides a similar set of features.

As you can see, on-line testing applications are very sophisticated and flexible. Not only can they be used in an on-line course environment, they also can be introduced in a traditional course where the students complete the test in a proctored computer environment.

CONCLUSION

On-line course development tools are becoming increasingly sophisticated. Course designers and instructors can choose between turnkey course development systems and general Web-development applications, depending on the needs of the instructor and amount of support and training provided. If the instructor chooses a general Web-development application, she or he can complement the course with a variety of third-party applications, such as a discussion board, chat, or assessment engine. Although many of these applications are relatively inexpensive, others are quite expensive and require technical personnel to install and maintain them. The best solution is to do careful research and adopt a standard system throughout an organization. This provides a consistent tool set for the course designers and students and facilitates improved support, as the technical team will be required to service only one application set.

REFERENCE

Robson, R. (1999, June). *WWW-based Course Support Systems: The First Generation.* Paper presented at ED Media Seminar, Seattle, Washington.

4

Clinical Applications of Electronic Learning Systems

Shirley M. Moore and Stefanie J. Kelley

The time has come to move beyond thinking of computers as assisting only with classroom learning or the acquisition of didactic content for nursing students. Computers also can be used by students to achieve clinical objectives. Clinical simulations and direct delivery of nursing care to clients by means of computers are two ways that faculty can use electronic systems to support clinical learning objectives. There are several reasons that faculty should use electronic learning systems to support the acquisition of clinical objectives of nursing students. First, content necessary for clinical objectives is overloaded by the amount of expanding health care information. Second, student access to patients through electronic hookup provides expanded opportunities to learn additional assessment, screening, and monitoring skills; enhance their teaching-learning skills; and apply interventions such as the provision of information, assistance with decision making, and emotional support. Also, the availability of sufficient numbers of primary care placement sites and adequate supervision of students in clinical sites are often problematic.

Another reason to expand our use of electronic learning to achieve clinical objectives is the increased opportunity for our students to learn about interdisciplinary care. Electronic systems can be used to access clients who can be cared for by an interdisciplinary team of students, thereby overcoming some of the traditional problems of getting students from different disciplines together at the same time and place to plan and implement interdisciplinary care. The use of electronic learning systems can also meet students' needs for more convenience in educational experiences by bridging geographic distances. Finally, we need to consider the use of electronic systems for the delivery of health care because our clients are using computers to access health care. In the United States the number of people searching for health information on-line is expanding, from less than 8 million in 1995 to an estimated 30 million in 2000 (Ghitis, 1999). With the advent of WebTV, accessing Internet health care resources has become financially feasible and easy to do. We must prepare the next generation of health care providers to develop therapeutic relationships by means of computers and to apply nursing assessment, diagnosis, and treatment.

CLINICAL SIMULATIONS USING COMPUTERS

Assessment and diagnostic reasoning are central to the clinical components of nursing curricula. Nursing curricula traditionally have been dependent on time, location, and faculty-paced instruction. Traditional classrooms are located in set rooms, at set times, with a fixed-pace instruction. Clinical courses have held tight to the paradigm that person (patient)–present education is the most effective method to educate nurses. The length of classroom time and the unpredictable exposure in clinical environments, however, restrict continuous reinforcement of assessment and clinical skills. Also, the nursing curriculum is becoming overloaded by the quantity of information from health care research. While students are experiencing the sticker shock of 25% increase in college tuition in the past 10 years, schools cannot afford to increase minimum credits in order to cover content (Wian, 1997). Technology, however, is allowing education to move beyond correspondence classes and the traditional classroom curriculum. Electronic tools can augment the learning objectives to better prepare the student for clinical skill acquisition.

ASSESSMENT SKILLS

Assessment coursework has traditionally been limited to classroom lecture and the laboratory with student partners. On-site demonstration and return demonstration allow students to build confidence in assessment skills. However, learning these skills is not exclusive to the classroom. The capability exists for students to study assessment techniques from a virtual classroom. For example, students can observe normal and abnormal anatomy from licensed software or CD-ROM or on the Internet. ADAM® software is available on the Internet for an access charge, or a CD-ROM can be purchased by the educational institution for student use. The virtual person, ADAM, becomes a virtual assessment partner. This assessment partner is presented in vertical and horizontal images, in which body systems have specific anatomical images. Students can use this learning program to better comprehend anatomy and physiology and learn beyond traditional lab experiences. For instance, visualizing the liver and surrounding structures enhances assessment skills by better preparing the student to palpate, percuss, and measure liver span.

Another electronic assessment program is The Virtual Body (http://www.nlm.nih.gov/research/visible/). This program is a Web-based, fee-for-service program funded by the National Institutes of Health. Male and female images taken from computerized tomography (CT) and magnetic resonance imaging (MRI) represent a 3-D human body. Exposure to diverse images of the Virtual Body add to a student's assessment skills without relying on lab partners or patients in clinical settings. Faculty can require students to submit assessment documentation from assigned reviews of body systems by E-mail. Faculty can electronically evaluate student documentation of assessment findings and review the student's comprehension, synthesis, and assessment skills. Although students do not have the ability to palpate the enlarged liver, the Virtual Body brings assessment skills to the student's location and complements the traditional assessment lab.

The virtual laboratory also can come to life with the sights and sounds of physical assessment by using computer .wav files. These sound files become virtual stethoscopes. The chance of auscultating an S3 or murmur on a student lab partner or rales and rhonchi during hospital clinical service is unpredictable. The computer becomes an assessment classmate. With a click of a mouse a student can auscultate the apex of the heart and compare it to the aortic sounds by using preprogrammed .wav files. The student can also use the virtual fingers to percuss the abdomen, assessing organ location by listening to resonance, tympany, or dullness of the virtual body. Coupled with the 3-D computer animation files from plug-in capabilities, students can then visualize the abdomen by taking a 180° trip around the abdomen observing peristalsis or aortic pulsations.

Other animated examinations use a mouse to assist the beginning practitioner to use an ophthalmoscope. The student guides the mouse to visualize the macula and optic disk as if looking through the small ophthalmoscope light to better understand the anatomy of the orbit. Another use of computers to enhance technical expertise is the CathSim® (HT Medical, Rockville, MD). Students can practice skills by using CathSim's animated computer program that implements specialized virtual reality technology to simulate intravenous (IV) catheter access. Students review a case, virtually prep the IV site, select the catheter, then virtually insert the catheter. The sights, sounds, and virtual touch of the software add to the clinical simulation.

Clinical education is further enhanced with the integration of live Internet access to classroom lecture material. For example, electrocardiogram assessment becomes easier to present when live from the World Wide Web (Web). Using images, audio, or video from the Web during physical assessment, didactic presentations can eliminate the poor quality of overhead transparencies and enhance students' exposure to quality ECG rhythm strips, often difficult to access in the clinical setting. Another way to enhance didactic presentations using live Internet access is microscopic slide gifs from the National Library of Medicine's Web site. Observing microscopic cells projected on a large screen live from the Web offers greater understanding of the smallest unit of physical assessment. Exposing students to Web sites in class allows the students to move the lab to the students' desktop at home and allows the assessment skills to be practiced in an interactive computer Web site.

DIAGNOSTIC REASONING

A virtual clinical laboratory for nursing students allows students to hone their diagnostic reasoning skills electronically. The expert model in nursing education adds to the complexity of learning and applying diagnostic knowledge. The National Council of State Boards of Nursing has been studying the development of a computer program that assists students to acquire diagnostic reasoning skills. The Clinical Simulation Test (CST®) is software programmed to simulate decision-making activities through case studies (Bersky & Krawczak, 1995). The use of case studies requires students to apply refined skills and pushes the students to be specific in their assessment techniques. CST is an uncued mock assessment lab. It is uncued in that it gives students the freedom to explore assessment techniques while receiving feedback on their performance from a database of default responses. The CST case studies enhance students' exposure to specific cultural, clinical, and disease-specific pathology that may be unavailable in the clinical site.

There are several Internet sites that offer case studies and laboratory challenges for further diagnostic reasoning practice. Medscape (http://www.medscape.com) offers bimonthly case studies. Faculty can require students to submit critical thought questions or diagnostic reasoning responses to Medscape cases. Students can explore the uncertainties of assessment and differential diagnosis in a safe environment outside the classroom or clinical arena. Part of expanding diagnostic skills includes choosing and interpreting laboratory tests. The Virtual Hospital (http://www.vh.org/) offers radiological and CT scan cases with diagnostic explanations supported by assessment findings.

Clinical exposure to specialty assessment and diagnostic skills is dependent on access to clinics and patients, which are not always available. Web-based learning can increase student exposure to uncommon problems. The Virtual Hospital's dermatology page (http://www.vh.org/Providers/Lectures/PietteDermatology/BasicDermatology.html) references dermatology in full text, quality photographs. This Web page supplements the students' clinical experiences by exposing common and uncommon dermatologic conditions. Pediatric patients present with a vast array of problems that can be difficult to decipher. Pedbase (http://www.icondata.com/health/pedbase/index.htm) has a database of over 550 childhood illnesses. This database can be accessed on-line or downloaded as shareware for students tackling the multitude of pediatric diagnoses. Additional virtual pediatric clinical experiences can be found at http://www.people.virginia.edu/~smb4v/casemenu.html. Students are given brief descriptions of cases and have the opportunity to reason the answers diagnostically.

To promote the diagnostic reasoning process, faculty can organize groups of students to confidentially post challenging cases on the course Internet bulletin board. Class colleagues respond to the posed cases by requesting additional assessment data, proposing laboratory data requests, suggesting diagnoses, and developing plans of care. The students who develop the posed case respond to questions and make follow-up recommendations while faculty monitor the progress. Students can respond on the bulletin board using aliases instead of their real names. The computer allows the student to "make a wild guess" without feeling stupid. This confidential and safe environment promotes students' confidence in their assessment and diagnostic skills.

Electronic clinical learning has the potential to allow greater exploration in diagnostic reasoning through electronically posed clinical challenges. As educators, our ability to have students interact with sufficient numbers of patients with unusual chief concerns in their clinical placements is a challenge. Web resources are a compromise to learning by using the live patient, yet they are complementary and include useful features to promote student clinical confidence, such as anonymity, self-paced learning, and freedom from fear of making a mistake on a real patient.

FACULTY CONSULTATION

A supportive electronic clinical environment for learning can be developed through several approaches. Traditionally, postclinical conferences were one-to-one or small-group opportunities to assess students' progress and reflect after a day in the clinical setting. E-mail offers the ability to conduct virtual postclinical conferences. In particular, faculty consultation and evaluation can be challenging for advanced practice nursing students in distant clinical practicum sites. Weekly E-mails between the student and faculty, as well as between the preceptor and faculty, allow greater contact and support. A structured electronic evaluation that documents clinical progress, patient contacts, differential diagnoses, challenges, and objectives achieved organizes the virtual clinical conference without struggling to coordinate time zones and distance.

Faculty can moderate course electronic bulletin boards to facilitate faculty consultation and provide student feedback. These bulletin boards can be anonymous, thereby decreasing the anxiety of posing a "stupid question." Electronic clinical learning experiences sometimes result in students feeling unsupported by faculty. Faculty can create a supportive environment by offering training sessions for students to learn how to individualize and master self-paced learning. Students need to be aware that the self-paced methods of distance or electronic education require an individualized structure. One researcher proposes a "meeting" phase during which specific time is set aside between the student and faculty to assess learning needs and to discuss clinical expectations (Lawton, 1997). As the student progresses through the course, a "guiding" phase occurs when progress in the course is addressed and future progression is encouraged (Lawton, 1997). These virtual meetings offer additional contact with faculty members and offer faculty an opportunity to more closely evaluate and mentor students.

DELIVERING NURSING CARE USING ELECTRONIC SYSTEMS

The computer is a new environment for therapeutic clinical encounters. Using electronic systems to deliver nursing care has been refined by the authors in a series of projects and is described below. In the first project, Brennan, Moore, and Smyth (1995) provided home care support to caregivers of persons with Alzheimer's disease, using a computer network, ComputerLink. Computer terminals placed in clients' homes allowed 24-hour access to a variety of features, including a communications module, an information module, and a decision assistance module. The communications module included a public bulletin board, where clients and a nurse moderator publicly posted and read messages; a Question and Answer section in which clients anonymously posted questions to a registered nurse; and a private mail system. The information system provided several hundred indexed screens of information about the disease course, diagnosis, and treatment; symptom management; care issues; and community services. The decision-support module guided clients through decisions, using an analysis process that incorporated their own words and preferences, thus assisting them to make choices consistent with their own values.

In this project clients with little or no computer skills easily learned to use computers and accessed information and support electronically. We learned that clinical interventions via computer networks require the clinician to have an understanding of how computer technology affects client participation, communication, relationship development, and group norms and both social and computer behavior. Several challenges of computer communications must be taken into consideration, including (1) lack of physical presence of clients, (2) diffuse time referents, (3) asynchronous communication, and (4) the necessity for clients to learn to use the technology. The absence of face-to-face visual cues requires the clinician to rely on a new set of cues, many of which differ from those of clinical encounters involving face-to-face or voice communication. Important communication cues are found in the content of written messages as well as in clients' uses of message spacing, word selection, grammar, punctuation (such as exclamation points and dashes), and the frequency and length of messages. Future clinicians must learn to recognize and use these new sets of communication cues to interpret both literal and implied meanings in their computer "conversations" with clients.

The diffuse time referents are a special challenge to clinicians applying therapeutic group concepts on computer networks. Diffuse time referents are present in computer communication in that space and time take on different dimensions than in concurrent discussions. Because of the asynchronous interactions (messaging back and forth over hours and days) of most computer communications, feedback on questions and comments occurs over a longer period than in synchronous communication modes. The inclusion of a date and time on all posted messages orients users. Clinicians using computers to deliver care must learn what constitutes reasonable response times in computer-mediated communication. For example, we learned that when facilitating a support group discussion in which clients are being encouraged to participate, a 36–48-hour waiting time between the posting of an idea and the responses of clients was common. Thus, analogous to "waiting out a silence" in a group interaction, the nurse moderator learned to hold her comments for 36 to 48 hours, allowing the client membership to participate actively in their support group.

The asynchronous nature of computer communication with clients is one of the most unique aspects of delivering nursing care by means of a computer. This asynchrony requires the clinician and client to include context in posted messages, because messages remain over time and are available to be read and interpreted in both near and distant future. Context can be built into messages by including references to preceding messages and by rephrasing questions or comments from other messages on the network that are pertinent to the discussion at hand. Another way to build context into messages is to use a title for a message that is consistent with the discussion. In the ComputerLink projects, each conversation strand had a unique title, allowing one to search and read all the titles making up a particular discussion.

Developing and maintaining relationships is a goal in any therapeutic clinical encounter. Several challenges exist to relationship building in computer clinical situations. In any therapeutic relationship, rapport and trust must be developed between the clinician and the client. When using the computer, "introductions" must be designed by the clinician. The introduction of new members is particularly important for group interventions. On ComputerLink, this was facilitated by having an introduction system that included a common set of shared information for all new members as they entered the network group.

Computer networks could be used by nursing students to interact with patients by answering messages daily, reviewing personal mail that might be sent to them by clients, and typing responses to individuals or groups. Under supervision, students could employ both individual and group interventions of support, information giving, encouraging expression of feelings and ideas, acceptance, reassurance, clarification, and interpretation. These interactions are done by typed messages and are asynchronous. Guidelines for the clinical use of electronic mail between patients and health care professionals have recently been published by the American Medical Informatics Association (Kane & Sands, 1998). These guidelines address such issues as suggesting turnaround times for messages, informing patients about privacy issues, establishing types of transactions (i.e., prescription refill, appointment scheduling), and use of names and identification numbers.

In another project (Moore, in press) interdisciplinary teams of students (medical, nursing, nutrition, management, epidemiology) work with an electronic community of individuals to change cardiac risk factors. As part of an interdisciplinary course in quality improvement, students (1) develop a therapeutic relationship with clients over a computer network, (2) assess clients' current health patterns regarding diet and exercise compliance with heart-healthy lifestyle guidelines, (3) coach clients to make self-improvements in health behaviors, and (4) track and trend data related to diet and exercise behavior over the project period. Using a self-improvement Website created by the faculty (http://www.csuohio.edu/hca/hca615/improve.htm), interdisciplinary student teams apply several theories of health behavior change, including the Health Belief Model, reasoned action, self-efficacy enhancement, stage of change, and relapse prevention. Clients are electronically "coached," using strategies of goal setting, benefits/barriers assessment, problem-solving skills, diary keeping, social support, buddy system, contracting, tailored messages, relapse analysis, and feedback. Students also apply principles of teaching/learning and electronic communications as they assist clients to change health behaviors. Students successfully conduct learning needs assessments with clients, implement strategies to change behaviors, and evaluate client outcomes by using on-line methods without face-to-face interactions.

Our experiences suggest that working with clients at both the individual and group level may be easily and well accomplished by using electronic care delivery approaches. Some challenges to using this electronic care delivery system for training students include obtaining hardware for electronic communications needed for Internet access and obtaining sufficient software to graphically display patient data to support behavior change. As a faculty, we need to learn more about combining and applying knowledge from the disciplines of health behavior change and computer science. For example, we are learning about the ideal client load that can be reasonably managed electronically by a clinician or team, how much electronic client contact should be done individually or in groups, the extent to which clients' families can be involved, and the correct balance between the amount of work done with clients on-line and using other forms of communication (i.e., telephone, written, or face-to-face).

Importantly, our experience has shown that electronic delivery of care to clients is a good way to foster interdisciplinary approaches to care. Electronic bulletin boards also can be used to support interdisciplinary clinical communication. Nursing students, medical students, and other health profession students can interact electronically and share discipline-specific ideas to clinical challenges posted. This approach broadens student exposure to different views of patient problems and interventions from multiple disciplines. The electronic bulletin boards can become a "pearls of practice" resource for students learning clinical skills. In our interdisciplinary course, in which students electronically interact with clients to change health behaviors, the interdisciplinary student teams hold virtual team meetings for case discussion of their client load. In these electronic team meetings, the students from the different disciplines share their own perspectives on the clinical situation and agree to the approaches to be used with the clients. Individual students of the interdisciplinary team take responsibility for being the primary electronic contact with a client to implement the team therapeutic plan of care. This virtual approach to team care by students has solved some of the challenges normally associated with clinical interdisciplinary learning in the health professions, such as finding convenient times to meet across different programs of study and finding a common client case load.

With the advent of WebTV, electronic communications with patients in their homes has become affordable, accessible, and user-friendly. WebTV (cost is approximately $99) uses a client's own television. In a recent project of one of the authors, HeartCare (Brennan et al., 1998), customized teaching and home management support are provided by nurses to patients for 6 months following cardiac surgery using home-based WebTVs and television sets. In this project, cardiac recovery information on the Internet was evaluated for accuracy, appropriateness, reading level, and gender focus. Nearly 200 pages of cardiac information not available on the Internet was created by the project team. These Web pages were entered into a database and are dynamically "pulled" according to a tailoring algorithm based on information about patient health status, gender, comorbidities, risk factors, and recovery time frame. Organized into sets of menus, the content presented to each patient is updated by the computer nurse modera- tor as the patient's needs change over 6 months of recovery. Following a nursing assessment at the time of discharge from the hospital, the personal pages are created for each patient, and they are accessed from their homes by using the WebTV system. This project, supported currently by the National Library of Medicine and the National Institute for Nursing Research at the National Institutes of Health, is an example of the future electronic patient care delivery systems that are being developed. Preparing nurses to apply the nursing process using this new medium is an important challenge for nurse educators.

INFORMATION ON THE INTERNET

As students begin to invite the Internet into their virtual classrooms and patients are reporting Internet heath care consultation, evaluating Internet Web sites has become an important skill for future health care profession- als. Students must learn critical analysis of Web site content, source of content, quality of content, and intended audience. The UCLA college library instruction notes the wide variety of Web offerings but stresses that not all sites are equally valuable or reliable (Grassian, 1997). Recom- mendations from the UCLA college library instruction (Grassian, 1997) suggest assessing the content and value of each site in comparison to others. Other guidelines encourage the users to identify the authors or producers of the sites and assess their authority or expertise to produce the Web information (Consumer's Union, 1997).

Students must make a commitment to critical review of Web sites. With this knowledge they will be better able to direct their patients to appropriate sites. Patients are inundated with Web Uniform Resource Locators (URLs) in lay press publications. However, frequent inaccuracies in treatment-related information on the Internet are prevalent (Bischoff & Kelley, 1999). *Consumer Reports* (Consumer's Union, 1997) has offered guidelines for lay Internet users to watch for medical fraud. When patients present information downloaded from the Internet, students should be prepared to analyze the information for accuracy and applicability. Also, patient education opportunities emerge to discuss proper patient use of Web-based health care resources and current treatment interventions.

Teaching patients how to use search engines, bookmark favorite Web sites, and access health-related support groups are examples of patient education skills that nurses soon will be providing on a daily basis. Nurses already are developing Web pages containing health information for clients. This is an important role for nurses because they are knowledgeable about how to tailor patient information to appropriate reading levels and about cultural and developmental needs of patients. Currently, many schools of nursing include Web site development in required informatics courses in their program of study.

CONCLUSION: CALL TO ACTION

Applying the clinical process (assessment, diagnosis, intervention, evaluation) by using electronic systems requires the traditional skills of clinicians, as well as new sets of knowledge and skills. Nursing informatics (use of technology to develop and evaluate nursing applications and processes that support nursing practice (American Nurses Association, 1994) are no longer optional content in schools of nursing. As this chapter has shown, electronic interactions facilitate the achievement of clinical skills for health professionals in teaching as well as achieving outcomes for our clients.

Nursing educators must make the commitment to use electronic learning environments in nursing curricula to prepare future nurses. The Joint Commission on Accreditation of Hospital Organizations (JCAHO) is mandating knowledge-based information systems to help the health professional staff assess, implement, and care for their patients (Jones, Wheeler, & Carter, 1994), and The National Advisory Council on Nurse Education and Practice (Department of Health and Human Services, Division of Nursing) has called for the addition of nursing informatics to nursing curricula. Thus, informatics skills are rapidly becoming basic competencies needed by nurses to provide quality care. Unfortunately, basic infrastructure for nursing infomatics is often lacking in schools (Gassert, 1998). Inadequate funding, personnel, and technology limit nursing schools' ability to thoroughly integrate informatics into the curriculum. We suggest that faculty use a series of small experiments (pilot projects) within existing courses to learn how to use electronic learning systems to support clinical objectives. Our experience shows that it is not necessary to think only in terms of moving a whole course to an electronic format. Rather, experimenting by adding an electronic component to a traditional course can be an effective way to integrate some of the advantages of electronic learning systems. This includes clinical objectives as well as classroom objectives.

In conclusion, future nurses must be technologically savvy to respond to the needs and inquiries of their colleagues and patients. The concept of a virtual clinical laboratory for nursing students will allow students to hone their assessment and diagnostic reasoning skills electronically. Electronic learning will not replace the one-to-one instruction in this practice-focused education curriculum. The electronic media augments the relationship between instructor and student. The valuable time spent between student and preceptor could be supported through electronic resources. What adds to the ease is that these electronic educational tools are time- and location-independent. Electronic learning transcends the problem of specific location and time restraints.

Innovative uses of software and the Internet and faculty and student participation to achieve clinical objectives can attract students from a distance or students interested in an innovative program that does not leave the learning in the classroom. Clinical tasks are coupled with faculty feedback by E-mail to support on-line student learning. Additionally, electronic evaluation and consultation of clinical progress adds to students' informatics skill acquisition and professional development.

REFERENCES

American Nurses Association. (1994). *The scope of practice for nursing informatics*. Washington, DC: American Nurses Publishing.

Bersky, A. K., & Krawczak, J. (1995). Building a nursing activity database for processing free-text entry during computerized clinical simulation testing. *Computers in Nursing, 13*(5), 236–243.

Bischoff, W. R., & Kelley, S. J. (1999). 21st century house call: The Internet and the World Wide Web. *Holistic Nursing Practice, 13*(4), 42–50.

Brennan, P. F, Caldwell, B., Moore, S. M., O'Brien, R., Sreenath, S., & Jones, J. (1998). Designing HeartCare: Custom computerized home care for patients recovering from CABG surgery. *Journal of the American Medical Informatics Association* (Symposium Suppl.), 381–385.

Brennan, P. F., Moore, S. M., & Smyth, K. A. (1995). The effects of a special computer network on AD caregivers. *Nursing Research, 44,* 166–172.

Consumer's Union. (1997). Medical help on the Internet. *Consumer Reports, 62*(2), 27–31.

Gassert, C. A. (1998). The challenge of meeting patients' needs with a national nursing informatics agenda. *Journal of the American Medical Informatics Association, 5*(3), 263–268.

Ghitis, F. (1999, March 19). *Popular health Web site begins offering information in Spanish.* [On-line]. Available: http://www.cnn.com (April 13, 1999).

Grassian, E. (1997). *Thinking critically about World Wide Web resources* (UCLA College Library). [On-line]. Available: http://www.library.ucla.edu/libraries/college/instruct/web/critical.htm (April 7, 1999.)

Jones, C., Wheeler, T., & Carter, W. (1994). The role of knowledge-based information. *SEA Currents, 12*(5), 62.

Kane, B., & Sands, D. Z. (1998). Guidelines for the clinical use of electronic mail with patients. *Journal of the American Medical Informatics Association, 5*(1), 104–111.

Lawton, S. (1997). Supportive learning in distance education. *Journal of Advanced Nursing, 25,* 1076–1083.

Moore, S. M. (In Press). Expanding information for clients: Using continuous improvement techniques to achieve health behavior change. *Quality Management in Health Care.*

Wian, C. (1997). *Debt 101: College graduates learn reality of loans.* CNN. [On-line]. Available: http://www.cnn.com/US/9710/23/charging.college/index.html (April 28, 1999.)

5

Focus on the Learner

Carla L. Mueller and Diane M. Billings

As nurses and nursing students increasingly seek access to academic and continuing education and require convenient times and places for educational pursuits, learning at a distance is becoming the norm rather than the exception. However, being a member of a distance education (DE) learning community requires changes in approaches to learning on the part of the student and additional services for technical, academic, personal, and career support on the part of the institution providing the educational offering. The purposes of this chapter are to identify the needs for learner support in DE courses and programs and to discuss strategies for providing the resources to support learner success.

LEARNER SUPPORT

Students enrolled in Web-based education face many changes that can have short- and long-term effects on their lives. Schlossberg (1984) reports that adult behavior is determined by transition, not age. Schlossberg's transition theory facilitates understanding of adult students in transition by providing insight into factors related to the transition to a new way of learning and use of technology. It can provide information regarding the degree of impact that the transition will have and the assistance that students will need to cope with the transition. Schlossberg noted that four areas influence students' ability to cope with transition related to higher education: situation, self, support, and strategies. Academic institutions can influence the *situation* by helping students to view the role changes initiated by college enrollment in DE courses as positive and helping students to manage stress. Faculty can influence *self* by facilitating students' access to psychological resources. Institutional support, computer training and opportunities for students to develop a support group via their DE courses can positively influence *support* for students during their transition to DE. To positively influence *strategies,* colleges and universities must have effective learning resources available to meet the needs of students taking DE courses for the first time.

Successful transition to DE, therefore, depends on learners being oriented to the unique aspects of teaching and learning at a distance. This includes informing the learner about the DE course; orienting the learner to the technology, use of learning resources, the DE learning community, and the role of the learner; providing technical support; and assisting the student to develop personal and study support systems.

INFORMING THE LEARNER ABOUT COURSES

Since DE courses represent a significant departure from on-campus courses, students must be informed that the course will use DE technology prior to registration (Harasim, Hiltz, Teles, & Turoff, 1996). Providing information prior to the course gives students an opportunity to determine if this course will be appropriate for their learning needs, to determine what resources they will need to acquire or access (e.g., purchasing a computer or locating the television outreach site) and to prepare themselves for new ways of learning.

DE may not be an appropriate option for every student, and providing students an opportunity to assess their own needs and learning styles may alert them to their own ability to be successful. Additionally, DE courses involve active learning, participation, and assignments that involve writing. Potential students may find it helpful to be informed of the demands of the DE course before they enroll. The Distance Learning Technologies Group has developed a self-evaluation for potential on-line students that can help students decide if a Web-based program is for them. Questions include "Do you feel that high quality learning can take place without going to a traditional educational facility? Are you a self-motivated and self-disciplined person? Are you comfortable communicating in writing?" (Bedore, Bedore, & Bedore, 1998, p. 17). A questionnaire entitled "Are

Telecourses for You?" is also available on-line at http://www.pbs.org/ adultlearning/als/college/quiz.htm and may help students assess how well DE courses fit their needs.

Several strategies can be used to inform the learner about the DE course, such as including the information in the university bulletin of courses, providing information on the school of nursing Web site, and mailing or E-mailing information letters. Some schools use a learner assessment, posted on the school Web site, which prospective students can use to determine if they have the technical skills (particularly computer literacy), educational background, readiness for the self-directed learning and independence needed for success in DE courses, family and employer support, and the time required for the course.

At the beginning of any new DE program it is helpful to use more than one strategy to keep the student informed about the DE options. For example, Cobb and Mueller (1998) found that although students had been informed about computer literacy requirements in the course bulletin, a follow-up letter was helpful in giving them further information and giving times of classes that students could take to increase their skill level.

ORIENTING LEARNERS TO DE

A comprehensive orientation program is critical to the success of any DE program. The type of orientation will depend on the learner, the course content, and the DE delivery system used, but in general it should include orientation to the technology, how to access and use the learning resources required in the curriculum, the norms of the learning community, and strategies for successful learning.

Orientation to the Technology

The use of DE technology, particularly TV and Internet, requires special orientation to the technology tools, course management hardware and software, and other specific skills, such as using a videocamera, sending E-mail attachments, copying to the clipboard, or using the course management hardware and software. Learners quickly must become self-sufficient, as technical support at the user site may or may not be readily accessible. For TV-based DE courses this may involve learning how to establish the network connections and how to use the cameras at the reception site; for Internet-based courses this includes learning the use of the computer, browser, Internet service provider, and the course management software and hardware.

There are several approaches to orienting students to DE technology, and the selection of the approach should be based on the needs of the learners. The most effective way to orient learners is in a hands-on immersion course of 4 to 6 hours (Harasim et al., 1996). This can be accomplished by having an orientation day on campus or at designated outreach sites. Others use TV technology or Internet chats to have all students together for the orientation. However, with learners geographically dispersed, it may not be feasible to have students come to a central location, and other strategies can be used.

Printed information that requires the least technological sophistication to send and use may be most appealing for some learners. The use of technology can be explained in user guides or handbooks illustrated with diagrams of equipment or sample computer screen views. User guides can be posted on the Web site. It is also helpful to have a practice course set up where students can test the hardware and software before the course begins.

Other strategies for orienting students to DE course-specific technology include using a videotape, CD-ROMs, on-line presentation systems, or streaming video and/or audio that demonstrates the use of the technology and provides orientation information. These strategies are more expensive to develop and deploy but may be helpful to students who cannot come to the campus.

Once students are oriented to the use of the DE technology, it may take as long as two to four class sessions for students to achieve sufficient skill proficiency to shift their primary focus to the content of the course. Faculty must be aware of the time it is taking students to be comfortable with the technology and should structure course activities that encourage both the development of technology skills and the acquisition and application of course concepts.

Orientation to the Norms for Participating in a DE Learning Community

As in any classroom, faculty and students establish the norms for appropriate behavior that facilitates participation and collegiality in the learning community. Norms should be established at the beginning of the class and reviewed and monitored as the course progresses. Norms include establishing and maintaining a sense of community, encouraging relevant participation, and respecting privacy, confidentiality and the ethics of the learning community. Faculty can serve as a guide to membership in the community by modeling these behaviors (Bonk & Cunningham, 1998).

Establishing a sense of community in DE courses is necessary to overcome the barriers of distance and technology and, in some instances, lack of visual cues (audioconferencing, some Internet courses, and one-way video TV-based courses). Community is established by introduction of all class members and if possible posting student pictures. Other group process strategies, such as creating a safe and supportive environment, encouraging participation from all students, and acknowledging responses, can be used to maintain the community (Harasim et al., 1996; Porter, 1997).

In Internet courses it is also important to establish norms for network etiquette (Netiquette). Basic Netiquette includes using student names, respecting differing views, being judicious in using humor, and avoiding insulting or hostile remarks (Harasim et al., 1996). There are several Internet Netiquette sites that explain norms for class behavior; students can be referred there.

Participation is critical to active learning for individual students and the overall success of the course, and students should be oriented to the nuances of using DE technology to enable class participation as well as to the expectations for scholarly participation within the course. For example, in TV-based courses students learn how to indicate that they wish to make a comment by dialing in to the discussion or releasing the "mute" function; in audio-based courses students must learn how to listen for appropriate pauses in conversation in order to gain the "floor" (Henry, 1993). Participation in Internet courses is heavily text-based, often using threaded discussions, which can result in large numbers of messages, and students should be oriented to posting relevant comments and threading them appropriately.

Because learning outcomes depend on course participation and collaboration, expectations for participation should be made explicit at the beginning of the course. These expectations may include minimum numbers of contributions to course discussions or specifications for role activities when working in teams. Harasim et al. (1996) recommend motivating participation by making it a significant component of the course grade.

DE courses are more public than most classrooms, and norms for privacy, confidentiality, and ethical behavior are extremely important to the success of the learning community. Both faculty and students are responsible for affirming how these principles will be used in their course. For example, students and faculty should agree to confine discussion of privileged information to the course. It is also important to protect privacy of clients and case studies that are discussed as examples of teaching points within the class; names and other identifying information should be withheld. Finally, school policies and ethical guidelines about use of published material, respect for copyright and plagiarism should be observed.

Orientation to the Role of Learner in a DE Course

The role of the learner is changing as the information technology tools of DE encourage active construction of knowledge, inquiry, critical thinking, reflection, collaboration, and use of learning resources and knowledge work tools. Students who are successful in DE courses are self-directed; independent; able to network with classmates, colleagues, and faculty; and are well on their way to developing the skills of lifelong learning (Harasim et al., 1996). Faculty can assist students to develop these skills by guiding them to identify their learning needs and consider how they will be met, by negotiating roles, and by aligning support from families, employers, mentors, and experts.

Although the use of DE technology may make courses accessible and convenient, it also transforms learning into active and collaborative experiences that may be even more time-consuming than that experienced in some on-campus courses. Course management strategies are necessary to assure productive use of time. Faculty can assist students in planning for adequate time for the course by specifying learning outcomes and the amount of time needed to attain them. Students should be able to allocate sufficient time for course activities, identify study space, and learn to use the technology before class starts.

In learning communities, students assume responsibility for their own learning as well as for the success of the group. Students may have to be oriented to teams and collaborative work groups; faculty should mentor students in the formation of productive work groups and monitor the development of group process.

It is also important for students to understand their own learning styles and how they might be affected when taking a DE course. There are several learning styles inventories available, and some are now available on the Internet. Students can use them to assess their own learning style preferences and assume responsibility for adapting them to the DE learning environment.

PROVIDING TECHNICAL SUPPORT

Although basic information about the technology can be provided during an orientation session, ongoing technical support is critical to supporting the learners and establishing successful learning communities. Technical help is particularly important during the first few weeks of the course, when specific problems with setting up technology and accessing the course are likely. Although technical help is specific for each DE technology, the course provider should provide general support. For example, there should be a central technical support center that is available 24 hours a day, 7 days a week. The support center must be able to assist students with common software and hardware problems and to troubleshoot and establish connections to the course during peak hours. Many technical support centers have a toll-free number, a pager system, or E-mail that students can easily access. Course faculty must be certain students know how to contact the support center.

Technical support personnel are particularly critical for Internet courses and must be able to troubleshoot problems with hardware, software, Internet service providers, and network connections. When troubleshooting, the technical support team should ask students calling for assistance what type of computer equipment they are using. Cobb and Mueller (1998) found that despite instructions regarding the type of computer equipment necessary for Web-based courses, some students chose to continue using their home computer regardless of whether or not it met the hardware requirements for enrolling in the course, and these incompatibilities caused problems for course access.

COURSE RESOURCE SUPPORT

Additional course resource support is needed for DE students. When students are far from campus, arrangements should be made with support offices to deal with DE students in some means other than face-to-face, or a special office should be set up to handle DE students. There also should be provision for phone or on-line registration (including drop/add) and advising. Support staff are the silent heroes of DE and ensure that the myriad details required for program success are dealt with effectively.

E-mail Accounts

E-mail accounts should be set up for students prior to the beginning of the semester. The university must determine if students will be required to utilize the university E-mail system or can utilize their personal E-mail account through their Internet service provider. If the university system is required, it must be determined how access to the system can be facilitated in a cost-effective manner for students who live outside the university local calling number. Faculty can obtain student E-mail addresses and set up a distribution list to facilitate communication to the class. Some Web-based courseware has a separate E-mail system set up within the courseware to allow students to have a separate E-mail account related to the Web course. This facilitates separation of E-mail and helps students who receive a large volume of E-mail on other accounts to find course-related messages in a timely manner.

Access and Use of Learning Resources

The use of learning resources changes in DE courses as students do not have easy access to the on-campus resources of libraries, learning laboratories, and other learning supports. Information about these learning resources should be developed and distributed to DE students to make sure that they are aware of the services that exist and of how to access them. Information about these resources could be placed on the Web and linked to a common site for DE students, or printed material about the services could be developed and distributed to DE students.

A wide variety of learning resources are available to DE students. Using computer-supported collaborative tools, students have access to experts, mentors, professional colleagues, peers, and a variety of faculty; and a host of virtual patients, simulations, case studies, and authentic learning experiences are easily at hand. Faculty can assist students by guiding them through this resource-rich environment as they locate, retrieve, sort, organize, synthesize, evaluate, and critique relevant resources.

When designing courses and learning activities, faculty must be aware of the limits of the resources and students' ability to access them. Creating options and alternative learning activities gives students flexibility in the choice of learning resources. Faculty and students also have to be aware of time required to access resources and plan for adequate access time within the time frame of the assignment or learning activity.

If the purpose of the DE course or program is to provide access and convenience for learners who are at a distance from the campus, faculty must consider differences in time zones, limits of local resources, and the extent to which the campus learning resources can be available to learners at a distance. In courses that span geography and cultures, faculty must also be aware of when holidays and weekends occur and how time differences will influence access to resources. Faculty also should determine whether current office hours and modes of contact fit the needs of DE students and make adjustments as needed.

Library Access

A single point of access to library services would guide students to available resources. As student-centered learning communities evolve and as increasing information is available on the Internet, learning resources are even more abundant and convenient. For example, literature searches, databases such as MedLine and CINAHL, and full-text articles are all accessible through the Internet. Additionally, many nursing journals are now on-line, often available through the school of nursing or university library. Faculty also can place links to these resources within the course or on a resource page of the school of nursing Web site.

Library access continues to be critical to enable students to complete the research for assignments in DE courses. Convenience proved more influential in the selection of a library to use than the resources that were available. DE students reported that they usually needed library resources quickly, with nearly 80% needing material within 1 week (Butler, 1997). DE students may never be on campus or may be on campus in a limited fashion; thus, alternative ways of obtaining library access must be developed so that students can access resources in a timely manner. Both students and faculty lack basic awareness about the library services available to DE students; thus, it is critical that information about the library's services be publicized. A survey by the University of Minnesota Libraries (Butler, 1997) found that although most students reported adequate computer access, "these students reported rarely to never using these technologies . . . for activities related to library research" (p. 3).

Technical help in using the library via the Internet is particularly important. The library should be able to assist students with common problems and facilitate their obtaining the references they need to complete their assignments. Many libraries utilize a toll-free number and supplement telephone assistance with E-mail to facilitate student communication during hours the library is not open. After-hours reference service options (i.e., automated answering of frequently answered questions and automated fax-back services for delivery of library user guides) also can be used.

One approach to assuring that students have access to learning resources is to place articles, reprints of book chapters, or diagrams in a course handbook that students can order through the mail. There are services that will obtain copyright clearance for these resources. Students prefer having required readings readily accessible and are willing to pay for the convenience of having a packet of required course resources. Another approach is to place all assigned readings on electronic reserve in the library. Electronic reserve would allow students enrolled in the course to have computer access to the assigned readings. However, 80%–90% of library materials remain available only in print format because of copyright issues and cost. Thus, it is still necessary to support delivery of print materials to students as well as providing access to electronic reserves (Butler, 1997).

Bookstore Access

The campus bookstore should arrange for DE students to obtain the necessary textbooks. Bookstore staff can make up a list of required textbooks that are accessible via the Web or can be mailed to students. Student ordering of textbooks could be handled via the Web or mail and books shipped to students prior to the beginning of the semester. Bookstore personnel should be available to answer questions to assist students during expanded hours prior to the beginning of the semester, to serve the needs of working students and students from different geographic locations.

SOCIAL SPACES

Teaching and learning are social activities, and faculty and students have an experience base in traditional and face-to-face educational settings where social spaces are well defined and assumed. In DE, however, the opportunity for interaction, social and intellectual discourse, and use of nonverbal cues changes dramatically. Faculty and students must establish different types of social spaces in order to overcome the barriers imposed by distance.

Facilitating Student Interaction

Establishing a sense of community in DE courses is necessary to overcome the barriers of distance and technology and, in some instances, lack of visual cues. Cobb and Mueller (1998) found that some students had a sense of isolation from peers and faculty when enrolled in a Web-based course. Students enrolled in TV-based DE can be assisted to overcome the perception of isolation by allowing time for student and faculty interaction on the TV before and after class for questions and to provide an opportunity for networking. Virtual cafés and unmonitored chats can be set up for students enrolled in Web-based courses. Cobb and Mueller found that students enrolled in Web-based courses were overwhelmed about the high volume of messages on the course bulletin board. If personal chit-chat is found to contribute to this high message volume, a separate bulletin board for personal interaction can be established to redirect the flow of such messages.

Facilitating Faculty Interaction

Interaction with faculty both inside and outside the course is critical to learning. Recent work using computer-mediated collaboration tools indicates that cognitive apprenticeship models, socially interactive relationships between novices and experts to socialize students into a profession, evolve as students have increased interaction with the faculty (Bonk & Cunningham, 1998). Regular office hours also must be established to decrease students' perception of isolation from faculty. By using computer-mediated collaboration tools, faculty access can be more direct.

Office hours in a chat group or using a toll-free number can provide time for formal and informal discussion with faculty.

Changes in communication imposed by the technology frustrated students. Cobb and Mueller (1998) found that students perceived that communication via the Web was impersonal in nature. They reported that their greatest barrier was not seeing an instructor face-to-face. Schutte (1997) also found that students in a virtual classroom seemed frustrated by their inability to ask the professor questions in person. If faculty have a camera attached to their computer software, such as NetMeeting, this will support transmission of images as well as voices. This visual enhancement is important to some students and may provide more of a feeling of meeting with the professor in person.

ASSISTING STUDENTS TO DEVELOP PERSONAL AND STUDY SUPPORT SYSTEMS

Students who are learning alone require additional personal and academic support to overcome the isolation imposed by DE. Faculty can assist students to be aware of these needs, embed strategies for student support within the course, and provide suggestions for obtaining additional resources as needed.

Personal Support

One little-appreciated resource in DE courses is the support families and employers can provide. This support may be even more important than that provided by peers and faculty, and it affects students' persistence (Oehlkers, 1998). Pym (1992) found that family support is essential to student success in DE courses; it is also true that the family must understand the importance for "study time" on the Internet and be supportive to the student who is "in class" while at home. Billings (1988) found that in correspondence courses (which may have similarities to the isolation of Internet courses) students relied on family and employer support to overcome barriers of isolation. Other strategies can be used to assist learners in overcoming the barriers of DE technology, such as establishing outreach sites where face-to-face assistance is available if needed. Another strategy is to identify several students within the course who have used the technology in previous courses and ask them to be available to serve as peer "technology tutors." Or employ a student who is adept with the technology to assist as needed.

The workplace can be an important source of support. Students should be encouraged to talk with coworkers about their learning and also to discuss learning issues applicable to their work situation in the DE classroom. Students reported that when coworkers were aware that they were taking classes they asked how the classes were going and volunteered to switch shifts near the time when papers were due and exams were scheduled (Oehlkers, 1998). Oehlkers also found that some employers provided tuition assistance, whereas supervisors were sabotaging students with work schedules that conflicted with their courses. He suggests that educators collaborate with employers for mutual benefit and learner support.

Course Study Support

Another type of support that students may need is assistance with the course content and in learning the content and skills of the course. Course tutors may be assigned to courses where students can be anticipated to have difficulty. Course tutors can be students from a previous course, a teaching assistant with the content knowledge of the course, or nurses in the community who can serve as study mentors. These supports may be based at a learning outreach center, collaborative campus site, or clinical agency, or through the use of the technology the tutor may have time on air or within the Web-based courses. The role of the tutor may vary from course to course and can involve assisting students to learn the content of the course and to develop writing or math skills or serving as a role model. Having study tutors in DE courses is particularly important if course completion rates have been low, if students have difficulty with course concepts or if they do not have well-developed prerequisite course skills such as language proficiency.

Peer study groups are another support for students. These groups may form spontaneously or with direction from the course faculty. Study groups can form at outreach centers or employment settings when a cohort of students is enrolled in a program. In televised courses, faculty can allocate time for small groups to work together. The Internet offers faculty an easy way for students to work together by using E-mail or a separate "chat room" or "bulletin board" established for this purpose within a Web-based course.

ESTABLISHING A STUDENT-CENTERED DE LEARNING COMMUNITY

The ultimate support for the learner is a course designed to encourage learning by taking advantage of the particular distance-delivery technology, as well as faculty who are prepared to serve as guides, coaches, learning mentors, and facilitators. Although there are specific course design and implementation strategies unique to each DE delivery system (Billings & Bachmeier, 1994; Harasim et al., 1996), years of research in teaching and learning have revealed seven principles of good education (active learning, respect for diverse talents and ways of learning, rich and rapid feedback, interaction and collaboration with peers, interaction with faculty, time on task, and high expectations), which when used consistently lead to effective learning outcomes and student satisfaction (Chickering & Gamson, 1987). These principles also are effective when used in technology-mediated courses (Chickering & Ehrmann, 1996) and can serve as a framework for choosing teaching-learning activities that guide students in achieving learning outcomes and personal goals.

High expectations are set through clearly defined course goals and objectives and negotiation of learning contracts within the course (Porter, 1997). Students in DE achieve learning outcomes as well as do students in traditional on-campus courses that use face-to-face instruction (Billings & Bachmeier, 1994).

Prompt feedback about the learning process, as well as outcomes, guides students toward learning goals and overcomes a sense of isolation. Feedback can be requested and provided by faculty, classmates, peers, professional colleagues, and experts. Faculty can support student learning by anticipating points in the course where students may require additional feedback and design activities to give feedback as needed.

Electronic collaboration tools used in DE classes also promote increased interaction with classmates (Bonk & Cunningham, 1998; Harasim, 1993). These tools promote group work, enhanced communication among class members, and formation of peer support groups. In fact, one of the advantages of DE courses is the richness of students with a variety of experiences and viewpoints. Faculty can encourage and guide this interaction to facilitate learning outcomes.

Active learning occurs when members of the learning community are socially and cognitively engaged in the course. Active learning aids comprehension and retention of course content, and faculty can design course activities that engage students with content and each other. Active learning is promoted through authentic learning experiences, by solving real problems, using problem-based learning, and developing meaningful products. Embedding these experiences in DE courses leads to relevant learning outcomes and contributions to the knowledge in the profession.

Respect for diversity is demonstrated by providing different ways of attaining learning outcomes, creating a climate in which there is respect for different cultures and viewpoints, and providing options for using a variety of learning styles. Faculty can facilitate this respect and model it through course design and implementation.

WHAT DISTANCE EDUCATION IS LIKE FOR STUDENTS

As noted, being a member of a DE learning community requires changes in approaches to learning on the part of the student and additional services for technical, academic, personal, and career support on the part of the institution providing the educational offering. The learning support services suggested have been shown to provide a more positive outcome for students and to facilitate their transition to these new modes of education. Common problems noted during transition include student satisfaction levels, frustration with technology, feelings of isolation, and perception of increased time spent on coursework. However, the better the student support, the smoother the transition for students and the more positive the experience. This results in increased student satisfaction and increased student retention.

Swan (1999) found that students taking courses via interactive video systems were generally satisfied with the quality of instruction and believed that it was a good method for offering courses. However, when asked about the negative points of courses via interactive video, they responded that it was boring to stare at a TV for the entire class period, that they were unable to see everyone at once, and that sending papers away to be graded was problematic. Swan also noted that students reported a perception that all remote sites did not get the same amount of attention.

Wuest (1989) noted that there was increased participation and therefore increased attention to students at the studio site of an audio-teleconference class.

Students in DE courses identify communication with faculty as a problem and requested more frequent communication with faculty during the course, as well as prompt feedback on course assignments (Blakely & Curran-Smith, 1998; Reinert & Fryback, 1997; Sherwood, Armstrong, & Bond, 1994). Engaging students during DE has shown to be helpful in alleviating communication problems. Fulmer, Hazzard, Jones, and Keene (1992) noted that although students were initially uncomfortable participating in interactive video courses, encouragement facilitated participation. When interactive teaching strategies were used in an interactive video class, students reported feeling closer to the faculty and to the school (Sherwood et al., 1994).

Students continue to identify frustrations with technological shortcomings of equipment used with distance education (Boyd & Baker, 1987; Cobb & Mueller, 1998; Phillips, Hagenbush, & Baldwin, 1992). However, despite these frustrations, most students indicated that they would take another course via DA.

Ridley, Bailey, Davies, Hash, and Varner (1997) found that students enrolled in on-line courses cited the ability to reduce the negative effects of distance and scheduling as reasons for enrolling in Internet courses. However, even students who had a positive experience with a doctoral course in a virtual classroom on the Internet preferred to come to campus if able to do so despite the benefits of convenience and access with the Internet course (Milstead & Nelson, 1998).

Student attitudes toward DE vary in level of satisfaction from enjoyment to anger or dislike of DE courses. Cobb and Mueller (1998) surveyed graduate students who had taken a Web-based course and found both positive and negative attitudes. Students who enjoyed the Web-based courses stated that it was a wonderful learning tool. They commented that it made learning more accessible and reported that they liked the convenience of having class at home. Other students, however, expressed strong negative feelings regarding Web-based courses. Some of these students reported difficulty learning while using computers. Others expressed the belief that Internet courses were no more than correspondence courses. Several students complained that Internet courses only provided an opportunity for visual learning, and they reported difficulty in comprehending what they read on the computer. These frustrations were also noted by Schutte (1997) and Cragg (1994).

Careful attention to course design can help make Internet courses a good learning experience for students. Faculty should pay special attention to the number of learning activities that are scheduled and the time they take for completion. Internet courses require an adjustment in teaching style and pedagogy to maximize effective learning and ensure that course requirements can be completed in a timely manner. A number of continuing education offerings are available to introduce faculty to these changes in teaching pedagogy and help faculty to be effective in a "virtual classroom."

Cobb and Mueller (1998) found that students complained about the increased time commitment required for Internet courses. Students reported that "class discussion" via a bulletin board took a great deal of time, especially in classes with a large number of students. Students reported difficulty sorting through large numbers of bulletin board messages when they all were somewhat significant. Students in large classes found that they had to log on daily to keep up with content. This was an expectation for which they were not prepared.

The students' report that time spent on Web courses was greater than in a traditional classroom is supported by Schutte (1997), who found that students in a virtual classroom perceived that they spent significantly more time on course work than did students in a traditional classroom setting. Time constraints may be a particular problem for graduate nursing students because they are primarily female. Von Prummer (1994) noted that women enrolled in education placed greater emphasis on their family roles, which created role and time conflicts; whereas male students reported no role conflicts and mentioned being relieved of family duties and given uninterrupted time and space for studying.

Students reported a perception of decreased interaction with faculty and other students (Cobb & Mueller, 1998). This is in contrast to Schutte (1997), who noted more involvement among peers in a virtual classroom. He found that the highest-performing students reported the most peer interaction; however, peer interaction was built into the assignments for students in the virtual classroom but not for students in the traditional classroom. Cragg (1994) reported that computer conferencing allowed students to participate in discussions and schedule their own learning time. The group of students observed formed a cohesive, friendly group despite initial frustrations with the equipment. Campbell (1998) noted that women may have needs for support that differ from those of men because women more frequently talk about a discomfort with isolation and place a higher value on connecting with others than men do. Because of these differences, faculty must remain vigilant for difficulties with peer interaction in computer-mediated courses.

Cobb and Mueller (1998) found that this decreased interaction also affected perceptions of faculty accessibility. Students reported that, despite 24-hour, 7-day access to faculty via E-mail and the course bulletin board, it was very inconvenient, if not difficult, to seek help with problems. They were frustrated by having to wait until the next day (or week) for help. They identified that being unable to get immediate feedback on assignments or questions was a barrier; they wanted immediate input to know if they were on the right track.

SUMMARY

Technological advances in DE have provided a variety of delivery modes to increase access to nursing education. However, additional services are required to deliver effective DE to students and to assist students through the transition to these new modes of course delivery. Faculty who develop and teach DE courses must consider the need for these support systems, services, and resources prior to implementation of DE programs and monitor them for effectiveness. The student services support staff are truly the glue that holds DE programs together, and they influence student satisfaction and retention. Continued attention must be focused on what constitutes effective strategies for assuring the resources to support learner success.

REFERENCES

Bedore, G. L., Bedore, M. R., & Bedore, G. L. (1998). *Online education: The future is now*. Phoenix, AZ: Art Press.

Billings, D. (1988). Attrition from correspondence courses: Development and testing a model of course completion. *Continuing Higher Education Review, 52*(3), 141–154.

Billings, D. M., & Bachmeier, B. (1994). Teaching and learning at a distance: A review of the literature. In L. R. Allen (Ed.), *Review of research in nursing education* (pp. 1–32). New York: National League for Nursing.

Blakely, J. A., & Curran-Smith, J. (1998). Teaching and community health nursing by distance methods: Development, process, and evaluation. *Journal of Continuing Education in Nursing, 29*(4), 148–153.

Bonk, C. J., & Cunningham, D. J. (1998). Searching for learner-centered, constructivist, and sociocultural components of collaborative educational learning tools. In C. J. Bonk & K. S. King (Eds.), *Electronic collaborators* (pp. 25–50). Mahwah, NJ: Lawrence Erlbaum Associates.

Boyd, S., & Baker, C. M. (1987). Using television to teach. *Nursing and Health Care, 8*(9), 523–528.

Butler, J. (1997). *From the margins to the mainstream: Developing library support for distance learning.* [On-line]. Available: http://www.lib.umn.edu/pubs/LibLine/LLvol8no4.html.

Campbell, K. (1998). The Web: Design for active learning. [On-line.] Available: http://www.alt.ualberta.ca/presentations/learnchar/learnchar.html.

Chickering, A. W., & Ehrmann, S. (1996). Implementing the seven principles: Technology as lever. [On-line.] Available: http://www.titlgroup.org/ehrmann.htm.

Chickering, A. W., & Gamson, Z. F. (1987). Seven principles for good practice in undergraduate education. *AAHE Bulletin,* (3), 3–6.

Cobb, K. L., & Mueller, C. L. (1998). *Evaluation of graduate students in a virtual classroom.* Unpublished manuscript.

Cragg, C. E. (1994). Distance learning through computer conferences. *Nurse Educator, 19*(2), 10–14.

Fulmer, J., Hazzard, M., Jones, S., & Keene, K. (1992). Distance learning: An innovative approach to nursing education. *Journal of Professional Nursing, 8*(5), 289–294.

Harasim, L. (1993). Collaborating in cyberspace: Using computer conferencing as a group environment. *Interactive Learning Environments, 3*(2) 119–130.

Harasim, L., Hiltz, S. R., Teles, L., & Turoff, M. (1996). *Learning networks: A field guide to teaching and learning online.* Cambridge, MA: MIT Press.

Henry, P. (1993). Distance learning through audioconferencing. *Nurse Educator, 18*(2), 23–26.

Milstead, J. A., & Nelson, R. (1998). Preparation of an online asychronous university doctoral course: Lessons learned. *Computers in Nursing, 16*(5), 247–258.

Oehlkers, R. (1998). Focus: Informal support. *Distance Education Systemwide Interactive Electronic Newsletter, 3*(9), 1–3.

Phillips, C. Y., Hagenbush, E. G., & Baldwin, P. J. (1992). A collaborative effort in using telecommunications to enhance learning. *Journal of Continuing Education in Nursing, 23*(3), 134–138.

Porter, L. R. (1997). *Creating the virtual classroom: Distance learning with the Internet.* New York: John Wiley and Sons.

Pym, F. R. (1992). Women and distance education: A nursing perspective. *Journal of Advanced Nursing, 17*(3), 383–389.

Reinert, B., & Fryback, P. (1997). Distance learning and nursing education. *Journal of Nursing Education, 36,* 421–427.

Ridley, D. R., Bailey, B. L., Davies, E. S., Hash, S. G., & Varner, D. A. (1997, May). *Evaluating the impact of online course enrollments on FTEs at an urban university.* Paper presented at the annual forum of the Association for Institutional Research, Orlando, FL. Available: ERIC Document ED410871.

Schlossberg, N. K. (1984). *Counseling adults in transition.* New York: Springer Publishing Co.

Schutte, J. G. (1997). *Virtual teaching in higher education: The new intellectual superhighway or just another traffic jam?* [On-line]. Available: http://www.csun.edu/sociology/virexp.htm.

Sherwood, G. D., Armstrong, M. L., & Bond, M. L. (1994). Distance education programs: Defining issues of assessment, accessibility, and accommodation. *Journal of Continuing Education in Nursing, 25*(6), 251–257.

Swan, M. K. (1999). *Effectiveness of distance learning courses: Students' perceptions.* [On-line]. Available: http://www.ssu.missouri.edu/SSU/AgEd/NAERM/s-a-4.htm.

Von Prummer, C. (1994). Women-friendly perspectives in distance education. *Open Learning, 9*(1), 3–12.

Wuest, J. (1989). Debate: A strategy for increasing interaction in audioteleconferencing. *Journal of Advanced Nursing, 14,* 847–852.

6

Assessing Distance Education Programs in Nursing

Karen L. Cobb and Diane M. Billings

Nursing faculty and students have been using distance education (DE) technologies to establish access to academic and continuing education programs for several decades (Billings & Bachmeier, 1994). Considerable investment has been made by state legislatures, funding agencies, schools of nursing, and the faculty and students who have been pioneers in using technology in nursing education. In spite of the increasing use of DE, little is known about the returns on these investments—if desired outcomes have been achieved, what teaching and learning practices produce the best results, and how to best use DE technology. Answers to these questions have been sought by a variety of stakeholders, including accrediting bodies, commissions of higher education, academic institutions, schools of nursing, employers, and the students and faculty who are the DE users. As the use of DE in nursing increases, it becomes particularly important to assess and improve practices in order to produce intended outcomes. The purposes of this chapter are to discuss the value of assessing DE programs, provide a framework for assessing such programs, report findings from recent assessment studies of DE in nursing, suggest strategies for gathering information from stakeholders in various types of DE programs, and consider how findings from assessment can be used to guide decisions about best practices in teaching and learning in DE.

ASSESSMENT IN DISTANCE EDUCATION PROGRAMS

Evaluations may be conducted for a variety of reasons (Chelimsky, 1978) and may include conducting an evaluation for management and administrative purposes, assessing the appropriateness of course or program changes, identifying methods to improve the delivery of interventions, and meeting the accountability demands of various groups. The scope of the evaluation plan depends on the purpose for which it is being conducted. The primary purposes of evaluation of DE are to collect data for management and administrative purposes, to determine the cost-effectiveness of DE, to identify methods to improve the course(s) or the delivery methods, to identify learning outcomes of the students, and to meet the accountability demands of students enrolled in the courses, as well as other stakeholders.

A FRAMEWORK FOR ASSESSING DISTANCE EDUCATION PROGRAMS IN NURSING

Distance education is a complex and dynamic interaction of the use of technology, teaching-learning practices, and the outcomes enabled by the technology (Billings, 1997; Billings & Bachmeier, 1994; Ehrmann, 1995; Harasim, Hiltz, Teles, & Turoff, 1996). An understanding of DE can be facilitated by using a framework that identifies the component parts and their relationships. Several national groups are currently leading efforts to develop theoretical frameworks, instruments, and benchmarks that will guide assessment of quality, cost, and outcomes of technology-enabled courses and programs in higher education (Ehrmann, 1995; Ehrmann & Zuniga, 1997; Harrison et al., 1991; Johnstone & Krauth, 1996). The need for a consistent and theory-driven approach to educational program assessment/program evaluation has been urged by nurse educators as well (Applegate, 1998; Ingersoll, 1996; Ingersoll & Sauter, 1998).

Using a theoretical framework for assessing DE programs has many advantages for nurse educators. A framework guides assessment of outcomes and interventions taken to improve DE programs and informs judgments about allocation of resources. A framework also lends rigor to assessment efforts by guiding analysis of the findings of assessment of DE in nursing, identifying gaps in the research, and selecting appropriate variables for future study. Finally, using a common framework can assist nurse educators to understand the impact of the use of technology on teaching and learning.

The framework for assessing DE in nursing proposed here has been developed from models used to assess the impact of the use of technology and DE in higher education (Chickering & Ehrmann, 1996; Ehrmann, 1995; Ehrmann & Zuniga, 1997; Johnstone & Krauth, 1996; Harrison et al., 1991) and from a review of the nursing literature reporting research and classroom case studies about the use of print, audio, television, and the Internet to deliver basic and continuing nursing education. Themes emerging from the nursing studies were used to confirm the development of this framework.

The framework for assessing DE programs in nursing has three components (Figure 6.1), and begins with the *outcomes* that can be enabled by DE. Possible outcomes include learning (course- or program-specific); access; convenience; satisfaction; recruitment, retention, and graduation rates; productive use of time; preparation for real-world work; professional role socialization; and proficiency in using computer tools (computer literacy) and knowledge tools. The outcomes are facilitated by *teaching-learning practices* that include active learning, time on task, respect for diverse talents and ways of learning, high expectations, prompt feedback, student-faculty interaction, and collaboration among peers (Chickering & Gamson, 1987; Cobb, 1999). Effective teaching and learning in DE courses and programs are dependent on *faculty and student development for teaching and learning* as well as *orientation to the use of the technology and ongoing technical and course/program support, motivated and rewarded faculty*, and *access to learning resources and services*. The framework, therefore also includes these variables as influencing teaching-learning practices. The third component of the model is the *use of the technology*, including technology infrastructure and user support.

Although not included explicitly in the assessment framework, the *costs* of DE also must be considered in assessment activities. The costs of DE to students and education providers have implications for assessing the practices involved in each component of the framework.

METHODS OF COLLECTING ASSESSMENT DATA

Distance education requires modification of methods of data collection compared to data collection that is done face-to-face or on-site. For example, in a classroom, a standardized paper-and-pencil form can be distributed to students, either formatively or summatively, to gather subjective data

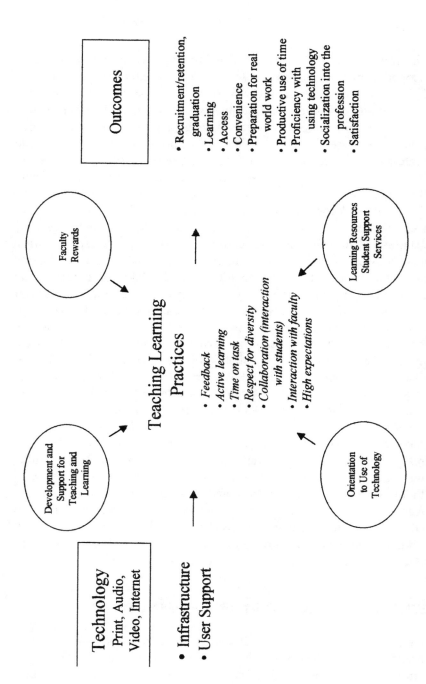

FIGURE 6.1 Framework for assessing distance education programs in nursing.

from students about the course and/or the faculty. Clinical performance data are typically collected by the faculty through direct observation of student performance. Exit or postgraduation interviews or surveys of either the graduates or the employers (or both) can be conducted to determine whether or not program outcomes have been achieved. Distance education courses and programs do not have the student on site; therefore, evaluation data often must be gathered by using other, more creative methods.

ASSESSMENT STRATEGIES FOR DISTANCE EDUCATION DELIVERY SYSTEMS

Depending on the type of DE delivery system chosen, a variety of methods can be used for assessment of learning outcomes, courses, faculty, and programs. As faculty move to the new paradigm (Barr & Tagg, 1995; Skiba, 1997) where the student plays an active role in the learning and assessment processes, DE courses must have a strategy for evaluating learning outcomes, courses, faculty, and programs. Besides multiple choice examinations, other methods to evaluate student learning include the use of portfolios, critiques, journals, papers, videotapes, audiotapes, "chat room" discussions, and simulations (Kirkpatrick, DeWitt-Weaver, & Yeager, 1998). Course, faculty, and program evaluations may have to be modified to fit the type of delivery system, as students are not on site in a classroom setting.

Print-based Delivery Systems

Print-based materials include correspondence courses, self-paced (self-directed or self-instructional) learning, and independent study. Correspondence instruction involves a set of preplanned, preproduced lessons conducted by noncontiguous communication, usually via the mails or through fax transmissions. Evaluation of student learning is accomplished through written assignments and examinations, which are typically taken by students in an educational setting near their home. Evaluation of the course and/or faculty is typically done after the final examination and transmitted by mail.

Self-paced learning involves preprinted, self-contained instructional units that typically focus on one topic (e.g., performance of self–breast examination). Evaluation of these materials and learning outcomes is performed by the student (Brunt & Scott, 1986).

Independent study involves a collaborative effort between the faculty and the learner to determine the student's learning objectives, learning experiences, and learning outcomes. Evaluation of independent study rests with both the student and the faculty and may be verbal or written, depending on the type of learning experience.

Video-based Delivery Systems

Video-based systems use either a television or a computer for instruction which is delivered by cable, microwave, or satellite on either open or closed circuits. Evaluation of learning outcomes may be done through observation of class participation, written examinations that are proctored by faculty at the reception site or completed and sent via the modem, peer assessments, and written assignments that are transmitted by mail, fax, or modem. Preceptors involved with students in clinical courses at various sites also may provide verbal or written feedback to the faculty about students and learning outcomes. On-site visits periodically by the faculty member can be used to decrease the students' perceptions of alienation from the faculty as well as for evaluation of student learning outcomes. Evaluation of the course and/or faculty may also be completed by the students with print-based evaluation tools that are sent via mail or fax.

Audio-based Conferencing

Instruction that is delivered via telephone lines through the use of voice and audio technology is referred to as audioconferencing. This type of instruction involves the use of two-way interaction from the origination site to other sites by way of speaker phones (Henry, 1993). Evaluation of the learning outcomes may be determined by audioconferencing participation or assignments or through the use of written assignments that are submitted via mail, fax, or modem. Student evaluation of the course and/ or faculty may be done via audiotape or through the use of paper-and-pencil evaluation instruments that are submitted to the faculty by mail or fax.

Computer Conferencing, Internet, and World Wide Web

Computer conferencing may include instruction that is offered totally via the World Wide Web or as a supplement to an existing course delivered by other DE methods. Computer conferencing "uses the computer to establish a network on a mainframe or file server in which an unlimited number of individuals can communicate with each other using personal computers linked by a local or wide area network or modems" (Halstead, Hayes, Reising, & Billings, 1995, p. 7). Learning outcomes can be evaluated through written assignments sent via the modem, written examinations or quizzes, and anecdotal records of the students' on-line participation by the faculty. Evaluation of the course, faculty, and technology can be completed confidentially by students on line using the modem (Cobb & Mueller, 1998), by mail, or by fax over the telephone lines. Meyen and Lian (1998) suggest that faculty and instruction offered via the Internet are subject to greater scrutiny by the public even if the course is restricted to students, and they propose that minimal standards of quality be set for Internet instruction.

FINDINGS FROM ASSESSMENT OF TEACHING AND LEARNING AT A DISTANCE

Nurse educators have conducted a variety of studies about teaching and learning at a distance. Findings from these studies provide a foundation for understanding best practices in DE and can guide subsequent research.

Outcomes

There has been considerable research and anecdotal evidence reported about the outcomes of DE programs. In general, program goals have been accomplished when DE is used as a way of delivering nursing programs; other benefits not able to be achieved in the traditional on-campus program have also been reported.

Learning

There have been innumerable studies of learning outcomes in DE in nursing, and virtually all studies reveal no significant difference when comparing DE courses with on-campus courses, using course grades as the measure of learning outcomes, regardless of the type of technology used (Bachman & Panzarine, 1998; Billings & Bachmeier, 1994; Clark, 1998; Fairbanks & Viens, 1995; Yeaworth, Benschoter, Meter, & Benson, 1995). Comparative media studies such as these typically reveal "no significant differences" in learning outcomes; thus, nurse educators can be assured that offering courses using a variety of DE delivery mechanisms will not compromise learning outcomes. In fact, when used appropriately, DE technologies have the potential to enhance learning.

Recruitment, Progression, Retention, Graduation

DE can be an important recruitment mechanism for schools of nursing and employers. Since the 1980s, video-based DE has been used to attract students who live near outreach sites that have television reception capabilities (Billings, Frazier, Lausch, & McCarty, 1989; Block et al., 1999; Boyd & Baker, 1987; Collins, 1987; Haggard, 1992; Maltby, Drew, & Andrusysyn, 1991). More recently, the use of Internet makes DE an attractive option for recruiting local, national, and global learners.

Although DE can be a recruitment strategy, benefits are lost if learners do not complete courses and progress to graduation. Several studies have pointed out that attrition can be a problem, and learners must be self-directed and motivated to complete a course or program (Boyd & Baker, 1987; Clark & Cleveland, 1984; Huckaby, 1981; Kuromoto, 1984; McClelland & Daly, 1991). Correspondence courses and independent study modules have had historically high noncompletion rates. This problem should be monitored carefully, as courses now offered by the Internet can have similarities to older forms of print-based instruction.

Graduation rates appear not to be adversely affected by DE. In fact, providing courses more frequently, compressing courses into less than semester time frames, and using other course scheduling strategies that are possible with DE (Kilian, 1996; Shoemaker, 1993), may shorten time for program completion and thus increase graduation rates.

Access

Using DE to provide access to educational programs, particularly in rural and underserved areas is a major reason that nursing schools and continuing education departments offer distance education programs (Block et al., 1999; Connors, Smith, DeCock, & Langer, 1996; Fairbanks & Viens, 1995; Sherwood, Armstrong, & Bond, 1994; Wieseke & Pavlechko, 1992).

The need for access continues to be important because many employers are now expecting academic preparation at the BSN level, certification is advantageous for practice in specialties, and continuing education is required for renewal of prescriptive privileges for nurse practitioners.

Several studies indicate that students are willing to overcome frustrations with technology in order to have access to educational programs that confer degrees, certification, and CE contact hours (Billings & Finke, 1998). In a study of graduate students enrolled in Web-based or total Web courses, Cobb and Mueller (1998) found that although some students had difficulties with the technologies used in DE, they were able to overcome these difficulties through assistance from the technical support staff as well as other students. Students also reported that taking courses via DE provided them with greater opportunities to juggle their course work with their family and work commitments. Siktberg and Dillard (1999) also reported that students enrolled in courses using the Internet expressed both positive and negative comments about this delivery mode. The students enjoyed the flexibility provided by this mode, but problems occurred when one or two students completed assignments in advance and had to wait to respond to a colleague's comments.

Convenience

Nurses are interested not only in having access to education, but as they place increasing value on their time, they are expecting to have education available at convenient times and places (Lowis & Ellington, 1991). With newer technologies that use asynchronous approaches to education, nurses can now participate in courses anytime and any place. For example, Cragg (1994) found that registered nurses in a post-RN baccalaureate program found "time-shifting," the ability to participate in learning activities at the learners' convenience, was a major benefit for taking a computer-mediated conference course.

Convenience also means that courses and educational materials are available for use at the work site. Television, computer-mediated modules, and Internet/Intranet technologies are ideal for making education convenient for time-pressed nurses and nursing students (Sheridan & LeGros, 1995).

Preparation for Real-World Work

Increasingly, nurses and students are seeking relevant, authentic, and real-world learning experiences. DE technologies have the potential to connect learners with simulated and actual clinical experiences. For example, simulations using databases, clinical information systems, and spread-sheets prepare nurses for the realities of practice (Gravely & Fullerton, 1998). Facilitating conferences on the Internet, developing teaching care plans, using clinical telehealth applications, or assessing real and virtual clients are additional examples of how learning activities and using DE technology can prepare nurses for the workplace.

Satisfaction

Student satisfaction with the experience of DE is important to faculty, educational providers, and the students themselves. When compared to similar educational experiences in the on-campus classroom, many students report general levels of satisfaction and indicate they would take DE courses again (Billings & Bachmeier, 1994; Billings & Finke, 1998; Block et al., 1999; Fairbanks & Viens, 1995; Kearsley, Lynch, & Wizer, 1995). Yeaworth and colleagues (1995) suggest that satisfaction is related to expectations of how the course will meet learner needs and is dependent on prepared faculty and functioning course-delivery technology.

However, not all students or faculty report satisfaction with DE. Several studies reveal problems with the technology as a source of dissatisfaction (Billings & Finke, 1998; Cobb & Mueller, 1998), and poor attitudes toward computers (Cragg, 1994) may cause dissatisfaction. Wizer and Lynch (1995) found that new students in a graduate program in educational technology leadership had greater difficulty both initially and later in the semester in the use of the bulletin board system than did students who had completed three or more graduate courses.

Parkinson and Parkinson (1989) noted that students reported differences in satisfaction based on having access to a "live" versus a televised faculty. Cobb and Mueller (1998) noted that some students expressed dissatisfaction with being isolated from the faculty as well as other students and preferred a live teacher in a classroom setting or at least via television. In addition, many students suggested that courses that are totally Web-based have occasional televised classes to distance sites to decrease their feelings of isolation. Hodson-Carlton, Ryan, and Siktberg (1998) reported that future graduate courses will include a mix of classroom and WWW delivery to decrease the students' perceptions of isolation and to provide personal contact with the faculty teaching the course.

Productive Use of Time

Distance education has the potential not only to make education accessible but also to save learners travel time to a campus or program site. Additionally, technology, particularly the Internet, can enable productive use of study time by providing access to course materials, learning resources, peer groups, experts, mentors, and faculty. Thus, study and learning time can more directly contribute to attaining learning outcomes. For example, Gravely and Fullerton (1998) report that students are more productive in an Internet-based course because they receive answers to their questions in a timely manner.

On the other hand, productive use of time can be diminished by technology failures that produce frustration and lost learning time. Failures in audio and television systems have been reported in studies by Billings and Finke (1998), Cobb and Mueller (1998), Boyd and Baker (1987), Phillips, Hagenbuch, and Baldwin (1992). In a televised course, videotapes and alternative plans should be in place in case of system failures, and course materials should be provided to the students well in advance.

Proficiency With Technology Use

One of the reasons faculty select DE, particularly the Internet, is to provide an opportunity for students to acquire skills using the DE technologies that are also the tools of knowledge work and clinical practice, such as search engines, literature databases, best practice standards, clinical decision-making tools, simulations, information systems, computer conferencing, telephone triage, clinical telehealth applications, consultation, and patient education. Recent studies report on the beneficial effects Internet-based courses have on improving basic computer literacy and competency. For example, Cragg (1994) found that students overcame their fear of computers and had improved self-esteem; McGonigle and Mastrian (1998) report that students' feelings of being overwhelmed and frustrated with computers decreased after taking an Internet-based course; and Bachman and Panzarine (1998) report that computer skills improve and also transfer to use in other courses. Kearsley, Lynch, and Wizer (1995) reported that students enrolled in a graduate course that uses a bulletin board system for communication perceived their knowledge of technology had improved and that they had increased competence and confidence related to technology applications. Older students or those who lack computer literacy skills can be introduced to technology through the use of E-mail systems (Anderson, 1995). Increased access to information and improvement in critical thinking and problem-solving skills, as well as enhanced participation through incorporation of the Internet, also has been reported (Sitkberg & Dillard, 1999).

Computers and the Internet-based technologies also have great power to enable the development of knowledge work skills such as enhanced communications, critical thinking, clinical-decision-making, and analysis of data sets. Wizer and Lynch (1995) reported that using the bulletin board system both enhanced the televised presentations and gave students a greater opportunity to communicate with each other as well as with the faculty. Harasim, Hiltz, Teles, and Turoff (1996) reported that on-line discussions among students were more diverse and deeper and engaged a greater number of learners in the conversation. Poling (1994) noted that there were increases in collaborative learning activities within DE student groups. Ribbons (1998) reported on the development of higher order skills of metacognition and found that an instructional database can serve as a cognitive template for clinical decision making. Todd (1998) reported that undergraduate students were able to improve their critical thinking skills and increase contact with the faculty member through the use of critical thinking exercises sent via E-mail. Students in Block and associates' (1999) study became competent in using videoconferencing as a skill for health care and consultation. Clark (1998) reported that many undergraduate students enrolled in a course with required E-mail assignments found value in learning the technologies in preparation for the computerized NCLEX-RN examination. Finally, as on-line communities of professional practice (Clark, 1998; Norris & Malloch, 1997) emerge, faculty and students will have increasing opportunity to generate knowledge in the profession.

Professional Practice Socialization

Nursing is a clinical practice profession, and roles are developed through mentoring, working with expert nurses, and establishing collegial peer groups and networks. Although DE has the potential to isolate learners from faculty, peers, and role models and thus decrease socialization opportunities, the research tends to show otherwise when specific strategies, such as chat rooms and peer mentors are used to overcome the barriers of distance.

Studies of socialization of nursing students in nonclinical DE courses offered by audioconferencing and videoconferencing indicate that students tend to form peer support groups and study groups. Having the faculty member meet in person with students periodically has also been reported to promote socialization (Boyd & Baker, 1987; Cragg, 1991; Reinert & Fryback, 1997).

The type of technology may make a difference to socialization practices. For example, Cragg (1991) found that students in audio-based courses were more easily able to establish peer support groups than those who were in correspondence courses. Although some students expressed feelings of social isolation (Cobb & Mueller, 1998), other studies indicate that students had increased communication with students who were geographically distant (Anderson, 1995; Wizer & Lynch, 1995). Cragg (1994) found that students in Internet courses do form strong bonds in on-line courses. Bachman and Panzarine (1998) also found that students in Internet courses communicated with their classmates and formed support groups that facilitated professional growth. Block et al. (1999) report that socialization and mentoring activities can be achieved by providing access to role models, peer support groups, cohort groups, and faculty mentoring through planned activities.

Clinical practice experiences are critical to professional role development and contact with role models. A variety of clinical practice models have been used to provide clinical experience in DE courses and programs (Block et al., 1999; Major & Shane, 1991; Viverais-Dresler & Kutshke, 1992). Some programs employ on-site faculty; others use faculty from the home campus who travel to outreach sites; preceptors and limited-cohort programs are other strategies. No difference in outcomes of these models has been reported.

Teaching-Learning Practices

In DE, the nursing classroom is no longer traditionally defined, and the use of technology requires changes in educational practices. DE changes classroom dynamics from an emphasis on teaching to a focus on the learner and learning (Barr & Tagg, 1995; Dolence & Norris, 1996; Skiba, 1997). The role of the faculty is to establish a learning environment that encourages students to explore and solve clinical problems. Faculty are content experts and instructional planners as they work with other experts such as instructional designers, graphic artists, Web programmers, and multimedia developers to develop modules, courses, and programs and select appropriate teaching methods and evaluation strategies (Bachman & Panzarine, 1998; Cravener, 1999; Hegge, 1993; Hodson-Carlton et al., 1998; Reinert & Fryback, 1997). The role of the learner also changes from passive recipient to active knowledge seeker as students assume responsibility for establishing learning goals and evaluate their own progress.

Seven principles of good practices in education have been identified which, when used consistently, result in student learning and satisfaction (Chickering & Gamson, 1987). These principles include active learning, time on task, collaboration with peers, interaction with faculty, rich and rapid feedback, high expectations, and respect for diversity; these principles also are enabled by DE technologies (Chickering & Ehrmann, 1997). The principles of good practices in education serve as organizing variables for the educational practices component of the framework for assessing the teaching and learning practices that are used in DE courses.

Active Learning

Students learn more effectively when they are actively involved, cognitively and socially engaged, and interacting with the content and class members. McGonigle and Mastrian (1998) established goals in their RN-BSN transition course on the Internet to promote active participation. When interactive activities such as on-line scavenger hunts that required students to engage in the learning process were used, the students' enthusiasm was high, and written work revealed attainment of learning outcomes beyond course expectations.

Time on Task

Learners must spend sufficient time with course content and participating in course learning activities to attain course objectives and outcomes. Several authors have reported that students spend more time in DE courses. Cobb and Mueller (1998) found that students reported spending more time in Web-based and total Web courses. Shutte (1997) reported that students in the virtual classroom spent more time on the class. Clark (1998) found that undergraduate students enrolled in a course that required Web-based assignments spent more time on the course content.

Feedback

Learning improves and is shaped by feedback from faculty, peers, preceptors, and mentors. Feedback is most helpful when it occurs in a timely manner and provides information about progress as well as process. Some students complained that it took the faculty member too long to respond to their questions and/or to read all of the messages on the bulletin board (Cobb & Mueller, 1998); other authors report that feedback using the technology allowed for greater access to the faculty and provided individualized instruction for the students. Anderson (1995) reported that the use of E-mail facilitated discussion that otherwise would not have occurred and that students could contact the faculty at times that were convenient for them instead of having to wait until class or regular office hours. Kearsley et al. (1995) reported that graduate students enrolled in an online course that used a bulletin board system cited the value of the assistance provided by their peers in the context of their class projects. In addition, students commented about the wealth of human resources and diversity of viewpoints provided by the bulletin board service.

Student-Faculty Interaction

As with other distance learning methods, students may experience a feeling of alienation (Cobb & Mueller, 1998); therefore, the faculty must find creative strategies for engaging the students throughout the course. This can be accomplished through the use of photos of the faculty member(s) and the students, access to the faculty at specified office hours via the computer or telephone, the use of E-mail to enhance communication (Todd, 1998), and the use of interactive videoconferencing occasionally during the course. Learning is promoted by meaningful interactions with faculty both inside and outside the course. In DE both students and faculty must strive to overcome the isolation imposed by distance in order to create opportunities for interaction. Interaction with television and audioconferencing is more spontaneous and direct and can occur during regularly scheduled course meetings; interaction on the Internet requires strategically planned time for one-to-one interaction. Reinert and Fryback (1997) found that students in televised courses have a great need to be in contact with faculty and to be assured that they are on the right track. Faculty promote interaction by having scheduled office hours, using toll-free telephone numbers, scheduling Internet chats or face-to-face visits at outreach sites or the main campus, or sending out newsletters or information packets (Fairbanks & Viens, 1997; Reinert & Fryback, 1997; Shoemaker, 1993). Other faculty who are using on-line instruction indicated that having regular office hours, either in person or via the computer, has been beneficial to students.

Interaction Among Peers

Peer interaction and collaborative learning activities also contribute to learning and satisfaction in DE courses, and faculty and students must assume responsibility for contributing to the success of the course by overcoming technical and geographic barriers. The use of student home pages, photographs, face-to face and on-site orientation sessions, chat rooms, and structured study groups are strategies to promote peer support. Asking students to complete assignments in teams is another approach to the promotion of collaboration, team building, and leadership skills (Kearsley et al., 1995).

High Expectations

Students learn best when they, faculty, peers, mentors, and social support systems (family, work colleagues) set high standards and expect success. Studies reporting the results of learning outcomes success and learner satisfaction indicate that DE does not detract from establishing and attaining expectations for success.

Respect for Diverse Ideas, Talents, and Ways of Learning

DE offers opportunities for creating culturally and geographically diverse learning communities. These communities are ideal for increasing global awareness, broadening learner perspectives, and developing cultural competence (Anderson, 1995; Kirkpatrick, Brown, & Atkins, 1998). DE also has the potential for providing options for learning and use of varied learning styles.

Development and Support for Teaching and Learning

When technology is introduced into the instructional setting, long-standing practices, traditions, and roles are changed. Effective teaching and learning practices in DE are particularly dependent on development for teaching and learning in the changed pedagogical and technical environment. Additionally, there must be technical infrastructure, access to learning resources and services, and technical support for the users. Finally, DE changes faculty work, and appropriate recognition and reward systems must be in place to support role changes. Development and support are equally important for both students and faculty.

Student Development

Distance education requires learners to assume responsibility for their own learning and to actively participate in course activities. Students also need orientation to the norms of the course. Specific strategies to prepare students for these changes are discussed in chapter 5, "Focus on the Learner."

Student Orientation for Technology Use

Students must be oriented to use technology. This can be accomplished by using student handbooks, posting orientation information on the Internet, conducting orientation sessions on campus or at the outreach site prior to the use of the technology, or using the technology itself during the first class session. Students are initially more uncomfortable about participating in class when using new technology, and they benefit from the time spent on orientation to the technology (Fulmer, Hazard, Jones, & Keene, 1992; Lowis & Ellington, 1991; Wuest, 1989). Billings and Finke (1998) found that technology training was not adequate for first-time offering of courses using videoconferencing and recommend more time be devoted to initial orientation. Cragg (1994) found that students' frustration with their skills in using the technology (in computer conferencing) was the biggest disadvantage of the course. Cobb and Mueller (1998) found that one of the greatest sources of frustration for students was a perceived lack of support when problems with the technology occurred. Students were particularly upset when assignments sent via the computer were lost or when their computer systems did not match the software program in use. In addition, students enrolled in televised courses at distant learning sites were particularly angry and frustrated when the system failed. Kearsley et al. (1995) reported that the most commonly cited frustration by students was associated with the telecommunications hardware and software to access the bulletin board system, especially related to file transfers.

Learning Resources and Student Support Services

Learning resources and student services sufficient to support the course must be available for students who are at a distance from the originating site of the educational offering. For example, academic advising, access to the bookstore, registration, bursar, and financial aid services all have to be available to students without their coming to campus. Additional services include learning assessment, career development, learning portfolio management, and competency testing. Of key importance is access to library materials, which can be made available at outreach learning centers or by using course pack preparation services that obtain copyright permission for required course readings. As the use of the Internet increases, to offer courses or as an adjunct to other DE delivery, on-line library and other digital learning resources such as databases, clinical simulations, and virtual patients must be available to students.

Most colleges and universities with schools of nursing offering DE courses have developed student services using the Internet or telephone to provide these student services or make arrangements to have them available at outreach sites (Block et al., 1999). Billings and Finke (1998) found that students are not adversely affected by having access to student services from a distance when on-line and dial-up registration services are available.

Faculty Development

Teaching in DE courses requires changes in teaching methods in order to make the best use of the particular technology. These changes may include adapting existing materials and learning activities for the DE delivery system (Major & Shane, 1991; Parkinson & Parkinson, 1989; Reinert & Fryback, 1997; Shoemaker, 1993) or modifying teaching style (Hegge, 1993). Teaching, particularly in Internet courses, changes the focus from an emphasis on teaching to an emphasis on learning, and because learning occurs through interaction with faculty, peers, and preceptors, learner-centered, constructivist, and sociocultural models provide theoretical guidance for selecting learning activities (Bonk & Cunningham, 1998). Making these shifts requires extensive changes to the design of learning activities. These changes are facilitated by workload adjustment and peer and administrator support (Reinert & Fryback, 1997).

Faculty Support for Course Development and Implementation

Overall, on-line courses have been found to be more time-consuming than traditional classroom teaching (Cravener, 1999). Developing courses for DE is increasingly becoming dependent on a team of technical and pedagogical experts. Content from an existing course often has to be redesigned and reconceptualized when the course is altered from a traditional classroom setting to a DE medium (Hodson-Carlton et al., 1998). Faculty need assistance with designing instructional material, using new teaching methods appropriate to the DE delivery system, and using evaluation strategies that can be implemented within the limits of the DE technology

(Yeaworth et al., 1995). Orientation to the use of the technology should include hands-on practice.

Faculty Workload, Recognition, Compensation, and Rewards

Faculty workload increases in DE courses because of the time needed for orientation to the technology and to develop new teaching materials, learning activities, and evaluation strategies; course development can take as long as two to three semesters (Fulmer et al., 1992). Various ways to support faculty are noted in the literature. For example, workload release time has been given to faculty developing courses for television (Boyd & Baker, 1987). Other schools provide teaching assistants or give additional workload credits, and some suggest that faculty who are teaching DE courses, particularly Web courses, should not have any other teaching assignments.

Faculty who teach in DE are also supported by rewards and recognition from administrators and peers to avoid feelings of isolation and marginalization (Shoemaker, 1993). For example, Billings et al. (1994) found that faculty in their study perceived support to come from administrators, telecourse staff, peers, and reception site coordinators; but interestingly, the highest degree of perceived support came from the telecourse technical support staff, and insufficient support for role changes came from administrators and peers. Recognition in annual reviews by administrators, positive promotion and tenure decisions, and merit and teaching awards are ways that faculty work can be recognized and rewarded, and they appear to be important for maintaining the quality of DE programs (Cravener, 1999; Monaghan, 1995).

Technology Use, Infrastructure, and User Support

The third component of the framework for assessing DE is the use of technology and technology infrastructure to support teaching and learning practices and to contribute to intended outcomes. The technology may include print-based instruction such as correspondence courses, audioconferencing, videoconferencing, computer-mediated conferencing, or a combination of several. DE technologies can be used to offer full courses at a distance or support on-campus course offerings. As DE technologies become networked, there will be increasing access to content, learning resources, and global health professions learning communities. Learning opportunities will be distributed, individualized, customized, and available at any time, connected to the real world of work and knowledge development/dissemination. Nurse educators must assess the technology support that creates the learning community and the impact the technology use, infrastructure, and support has on the educational practices and program outcomes.

Technology Use

Technology must be available to support DE. Technology must be used appropriately in appropriate combinations to support program goals and learning outcomes. Most important, technology must be reliable. Many authors report frustration and disruption to learning when the technology is "down," or not working optimally.

Infrastructure

DE programs depend on an accessible and reliable technical infrastructure. The infrastructure includes reliable service to the end user (home, reception site, outreach site, workplace) and easy-to-use communication and collaborative work tools, such as course management software, two-way video connections, electronic mail, and computer conferencing software. The infrastructure also must include the support personnel that maintain the technology or support the reception site (Billings et al., 1994).

User Support

When compared with traditional campus-based courses, it appears that planning, preparation and presentation of content, course design, instructional activities, and many other faculty activities are qualitatively affected by DE courses and programs (Cravener, 1999). Students and faculty need ongoing assistance for using technologies to offer DE courses, particularly when the courses use video or the Internet (Billings et al., 1994; Block et al., 1999; Cragg, 1994; Reinert & Fryback, 1997; Shoemaker, 1993). For example, in televised courses, user assistance is provided by technicians who manage the origination and reception sites, and in Internet courses a 24-hour technical assistance service should be available. Internet courses also use programmers to structure the course software, log students into courses, and maintain the file server.

Costs

One major advantage of providing DE is cost savings, especially when participants are willing to share the costs of the instruction. Distance education can provide a means for students to achieve their educational goals even though they live great distances from an educational site (Clark & Cohen, 1992). Cost savings also may be realized by decreasing learning time for the students and saving travel time and expenses to send faculty or students to remote sites. With certain DE strategies, students can continue to be employed, carry out their family responsibilities, and continue their education at their own pace or when it is convenient for the student (i.e., computer conferencing or correspondence courses).

Distance education delivery methods may, however, incur greater costs, depending on the method chosen for course delivery. Delivering courses via certain DE strategies involves additional financial costs as well as faculty and student time commitments (Reinert & Fryback, 1997). Cost-effectiveness must be considered when enrollment in a course involves only a small number of students. Whereas some universities and colleges may provide release time to faculty for course development and implementation, other universities and colleges may simply add this teaching assignment to the faculty member's already full teaching load (Cravener, 1999; Reinert & Fryback, 1997). Computer conferencing, which includes forums, chat rooms, and E-mail assignments, may provide one-to-one communication with students, but this can be extremely time-consuming for the faculty (Kearsley et al., 1995). Investments in technology can be expensive, and the educational consequences of this investment can be difficult to determine (Erhmann & Zuniga, 1997). If students must travel great distances to the course delivery site, both financial costs and time commitments can be considerable.

Several authors (Kearsley et al., 1995; Meyen, Lian, & Tangen, 1998) suggest that one of the advantages of DE is increased access to higher education, because instruction can be delivered to students regardless of where they reside. Although increasing access of students to instruction and other educational resources is a desirable goal of DE, it may decrease access for students who are financially disadvantaged. If financially disadvantaged students are unable to purchase the necessary equipment (e.g., personal computer with a modem), then access to the course and educational resources have been restricted unless they can locate a computer terminal. Long-distance telephone charges or local area providers for Internet connections also can impose additional costs. If there is a decrease in student enrollment or an increase in student withdrawals either because of access or financial issues, this will have an impact on the course(s) and the nursing program. Faculty, administrators, and students must all be involved in the decision-making process related to distance education.

Finally, there are costs related to the actual evaluation process that must be considered. Input from students takes time, analysis of the data collected takes time and may bear a financial cost, and there may be costs related to the decision-making process, depending on the data analysis. Analysis of costs versus benefits is an essential component of the evaluation process in any DE program.

ANALYZING, REPORTING, AND USING FINDINGS OF ASSESSMENT FOR DECISION MAKING

The primary purpose of any form of assessment should be to judge the merit or the worth of whatever is being evaluated, whether it be student learning outcomes from a course or program, the instructional activities of the faculty member, a particular course, or the medium used either as an adjunct or as a delivery method for a specific course or program. The significance of placing meaning and value on the data collected and that a judgment is made about the data are an essential point. If no judgment is made, then the basis for rational decision making cannot be accomplished (Applegate, 1998).

Analysis of the data collected "must consider not only whether the mission and goals have been achieved but also whether they are worth achieving" (Applegate, 1998, p. 424). In addition to the evaluation of student learning outcomes, universities and colleges often require evaluation of courses, faculty, and programs on the traditional campus. Distance education involves an additional evaluation component: the medium used to deliver the instruction. As in traditional campus classroom settings, data collected through the evaluation process for DE courses must be used for making rational decisions and ultimately involves faculty, administrators, and the various stakeholders.

Another essential component of any evaluation process involves reporting the findings and using the findings for decision-making purposes. The evaluation plan for DE should include a time line for communication of the findings to the appropriate individuals and determining when and how the findings will be reported. Confidentiality is an essential component of any evaluation report (Bourke & Ihrke, 1998).

Once the evaluation data has been collected and analyzed, the data should be available to the appropriate individuals for rational decision making. Bourke and Ihrke (1998) suggest placing the findings of the evaluation in context and explaining what the findings mean and how the results can be used. Depending on the data analysis, decisions may have to be made related to how to facilitate student learning, diagnose problems either with the method of instruction or the medium used for instruction, improve course or program delivery, and judge the effectiveness of a particular course or program (Bourke & Ihrke, 1998).

Other decisions that are inherent in DE courses and programs involve effective and efficient use of student and faculty time, faculty workload issues, promotion and tenure issues, merit raise concerns, ethical and proprietary issues (i.e., who "owns" the course[s]), costs related to course delivery methods, and student costs related to traveling to the origination or televised site, equipment expenses (computers, modems, and service provider charges), and mailing costs for submission of required assignments. Results of the data analysis should be used for strategic planning, such as appropriate use of faculty, resources, and recruitment and retention of students and should indicate a direction for improvement of student outcomes and course materials. Formative and summative student and faculty input should focus on methods to improve student support services, course revisions, content, and teaching-learning strategies. Based on the data collected, there may have to be decisions related to whether or not the program should continue using DE. Final analysis of the data should be shared with the appropriate individuals, such as administration, faculty members, and other stakeholders.

SUMMARY

Evaluation of DE is a comprehensive process that includes input from all individuals involved. As the use of DE in nursing increases, particularly with the explosion of Internet courses, stakeholders will demand that evaluative data are collected, analyzed, reported, and used for decision making. This chapter has described concepts related to evaluation of DE programs and has outlined a framework for evaluation of DE programs. This framework can be used to guide the best practices for DE and ensure that quality and integrity are not compromised when courses are offered via DE. The use of a framework also provides the "guiding force" (Applegate, 1998, p. 456) for ensuring the validity and reliability of the evaluation plan.

REFERENCES

Anderson, D. G. (1995). Electronic education: E-mail links students and faculty. *Nurse Educator, 20*(4), 8–11.

Applegate, M. H. (1998). Educational program evaluation.In D. M. Billings & J. M. Halstead (Eds.), *Teaching in nursing: A guide for faculty* (pp. 423–457). Philadelphia: W. B. Saunders.

Bachman, J. A., & Panzarine, S. (1998). Enabling student nurses to use the information superhighway. *Journal of Nursing Education, 37*(4), 155–161.

Barr, R., & Tagg, J. (1995). From teaching to learning: A new paradigm for undergraduate education. *Change, 27*(6), 13–25.

Billings, D. M. (1997, January). *Current status and future directions of distance education in nursing.* Paper presented to Division of Nursing. Alexandria, VA. National Institutes of Health.

Billings, D. M., & Bachmeier, B. (1994). Teaching and learning at a distance: A review of the literature. In L. R. Allen (Ed.), *Review of research in nursing education* (pp. 1–32). New York: National League for Nursing.

Billings, D., Durham, J., Finke, L., Boland, D., Smith, S., & Manz, B. (1994). Faculty perceptions of teaching on television: One school's experience. *Journal of Professional Nursing, 10*(5), 307–312.

Billings, D. M., & Finke, L. (1998, January). *Technology-mediated nursing courses: Students' perceptions of access and outcomes.* Symposium conducted by the NLN Council of Research in Nursing Education, Atlanta, GA.

Billings, D., Frazier, H., Lausch, J., & McCarty, J. (1989). Videoteleconferencing: Solving mobility and recruitment problems. *Nurse Educator, 14*(2), 12–16.

Block, D., Josten, L. E., Lia-Hoagber, B., Kerr, M., Smith, M. J., Lewis, M. L., & Hutton, S. J. (1999). Fulfilling regional needs for specialty nurses through limited cohort graduate education. *Nursing Outlook, 47*(1), 23–29.

Bonk, C. J., & Cunningham, D. J. (1998). Searching for learner-centered, constructivist, and sociocultural components of collaborative educational learning tools. In C. J. Bonk & K. S. King (Eds.), *Electronic collaborators* (pp. 25–50). Mahwah, NJ: Lawrence Erlbaum Associates.

Bourke, M. P., & Ihrke, B. A. (1998). The evaluation process. In D. Billings & J. Halstead (Eds.), *Teaching in nursing: A guide for faculty* (pp. 349–366). Philadelphia: W. B. Saunders.

Boyd, S., & Baker, C. M. (1987). Using television to teach. *Nursing and Health Care, 8*(9), 523–527.

Brunt, B., & Scott, A. L. (1986). Factors to consider in the development of self-instructional materials. *Journal of Continuing Education in Nursing, 17*(3), 87–93.

Chelimsky, E. (1978). Differing perspectives of evaluation. In C. C. Rentz & R. R. Rentz (Eds.), *Evaluating federally sponsored programs: New directions for program evaluation* (Vol. 2, pp. 19–38). San Francisco: Jossey Bass.

Chickering, A. W., & Ehrmann, S. (1996). *Implementing the seven principles: Technology as lever.* [On-line]. Available: http://www.tltgroup.org/ehrmann.htm

Chickering, A. W., & Gamson, Z. F. (1987). Seven principles for good practice in undergraduate education. *AAHE Bulletin, 39*(7), 306.

Clark, C. E., & Cleveland, T. L. (1984). The media and the mode. *Journal of Continuing Education in Nursing, 15*(5), 168–172.

Clark, C. E., & Cohen, J. A. (1992). Distance learning: New partnerships for nursing in rural areas. In P. Winstead-Fry, J. C. Tiffany, & R.V. Shippee-Rice (Eds.), *Rural health nursing: Stories of creativity, commitment and connectedness* (pp. 359–388). New York: National League for Nursing.

Clark, D. J. (1998). Incorporating an Internet Web site into an existing nursing class. *Computers in Nursing, 16*(4), 219–222.

Cobb, K. L. (1999). Interactive videodisc instruction with undergraduate students using cooperative learning strategies. *Computers in Nursing, 17*(1), 89–96.

Cobb, K. L., & Mueller, C. (1998). *Evaluation of graduate nursing students in a virtual classroom.* Unpublished manuscript.

Collins, F. (1987). Reaching out. *RNABC News, 19*(5), 24–26.

Connors, H. R., Smith, C., DeCock, T. S., & Langer, B. (1996). Kansas nurses surf Web for master's degrees. *Reflections,* 2nd quarter, *22*(2), 7–16.

Cragg, C. E. (1994). Distance learning through computer conferences. *Nurse Educator, 19*(2), 10–14.

Cragg, C. E. (1991). Professional resocialization of post-RN baccalaureate students by distance education. *Journal of Nursing Education, 30*(6), 256–260.

Cravener, P. A. (1999). Faculty experiences with providing online courses. *Computers in Nursing, 17*(1), 42–47.

Dolence, M. G., & Norris, D. M. (1995). *Transforming higher education.* Ann Arbor, MI: Society for College and University Planning.

Erhmann, S. (1995). Asking the right questions: What does research tell us about technology and higher learning? *Change, 27*(2), 20–27.

Ehrmann, S. C., & Zuniga, R. E. (1997). *The flashlight evaluation handbook.* Washington, DC: Corporation for Public Broadcasting.

Fairbanks, J., & Viens, D. (1995). What's happening. Distance education for nurse practitioners—a partial solution. *Journal of the American Academy of Nurse Practitioners, 7*(10), 499–503.

Fulmer, J., Hazard, M., Jones, S., & Keene, K. (1992). Distance learning: An innovative approach to nursing education. *Journal of Professional Nursing, 8*(5), 289–294.

Graveley, E., & Fullerton, J. T. (1998). Incorporating electronic-based and computer-based strategies: Graduate nursing courses in administration. *Journal of Nursing Education, 37*(4), 186–188.

Haggard, A. (1992). Using self studies to meet JCAHO requirements. *Journal of Nursing Staff Development, 8*(4), 170–173.

Halstead, J., Hayes, R., Reising, D., & Billings, D. (1995). Nursing student information network: Fostering collegial communications using a computer conference. *Computers in Nursing, 13*(2), 55–59.

Harasim, L., Hiltz, S. R., Teles, L., & Turoff, M. (1996). *Learning networks: A field guide to teaching and learning on-line.* Cambridge, MA: Massachusetts Institute of Technology.

Harrison, P. J., Seeman, B. B., Behnm, R., Saba, F., Molise, G., & Williams, M. D. (1991). Development of a distance education assessment instrument. *Educational Technology Research and Development, 39*(4), 65–77.

Hegge, M. (1993). Interactive television presentation style and teaching materials. *Journal of Continuing Education in Nursing, 24,* 39–42.

Henry, P. (1993). Distance learning through audioconferencing. *Nurse Educator, 18*(2), 23–26.

Hodson-Carlton, K. H., Ryan, M. E., & Siktberg, L. L. (1998). Designing courses for the Internet. *Nurse Educator, 23*(3), 45–50.

Huckaby, L. (1981). The effects of modularized instruction and traditional teaching techniques on cognitive learning and affective behaviors of student nurses. *Advances in Nursing Science, 33,* 67–82.

Ingersoll, G. L. (1996). Evaluation research. *Nursing Administration Quarterly, 20*(4), 28–40.

Ingersoll, G. L., & Sauter, M. (1998). Integrating accreditation criteria into educational program evaluation. *Nursing and Health Care Perspectives, 19*(5), 224–229.

Johnstone, S. M., & Krauth, B. (1996). Some principles of good practice for the virtual university. *Change, 28*(2), 39–41.

Kearsley, G., Lynch, W., & Wizer, D. (1995). The effectiveness and impact of online learning in graduate education. *Educational Technology, 35*(6), 37–42.

Kilian, C. (1996). An on-line writing course (article originally posted to the *Online Community College List*, January 22, 1996. [Available from Crawford Killian, Communications Department, Capilano College, 2055 Purcell Way, North Vancouver, BC, Canada V7J3H5].

Kirkpatrick, J. M., DeWitt-Weaver, D., & Yeager, L. (1998). Strategies for evaluating learning outcomes. In D. M. Billings & J. M. Halstead (Eds.), *Teaching in nursing: A guide for faculty* (pp. 367–384). Philadelphia: W. B. Saunders.

Kirkpatrick, M. K., Brown, S., & Atkins, T. (1998). Electronic education: Using the Internet to integrate cultural diversity and global awareness. *Nurse Educator, 23*(2), 15–17.

Kuromoto, A. (1984). Teleconferencing for nurses: Evaluating its effectiveness. In L. A. Parker & C. H. Olgren (Eds.), *Teleconferencing and electronic communications* (Vol. 3, pp. 262–268). Madison, WI: University of Wisconsin Extension, Center for Interactive Programs.

Lowis, A., & Ellington, H. (1991). Innovations in occupational health nursing education,including a distance learning approach. *American Association of Occupational Health Nursing Journal, 39*(7), 316–318.

Major, M. B., & Shane, D. L. (1991). Use of interactive television for outreach nursing education. *American Journal of Distance Education, 5*(1), 57–66.

Maltby, H., Drew, L., & Andrusysyn, M. A. (1991). Distance education: Joining forces to meet the challenge. *Journal of Continuing Education in Nursing, 22*(3), 119–122.

McClelland, E., & Daly, J. (1991). A comparison of selected demographic characteristics and academic performance of on campus and satellite center RN's: Implications for the curriculum. *Journal of Nursing Education, 30*(6), 261–266.

McGonigle, D., & Mastrain, K. (1998). Learning along the way: Cyberspatial quests. *Nursing Outlook, 46*(2), 81–86.

Meyen, E. L., Lian, C. H., & Tangen, P. (Spring, 1998). Issues associated with the design and delivery of online instruction. *Focus on Autism and other Developmental Disabilities, 13*(1), 53–61.

Monaghan, P. (1995). Technology and the unions. *Chronicle of Higher Education, 42,* A17–A18.

Norris, D. M., & Malloch, T. R. (1997). *Unleashing the power of perpetual learning.* Ann Arbor, MI: Society for College and University Planning.

Parkinson, C. F., & Parkinson, S. B. (1989). A comparative study between interactive television and traditional lecture course offerings for nursing students. *Nursing and Health Care, 10*(9), 499–502.

Phillips, C. Y., Hagenbuch, E. G., & Baldwin, P. J. (1992). A collaborative effort in using telecommunications to enhance learning. *Journal of Continuing Education in Nursing, 23*(3), 134–138.

Poling, D. J. (1994). E-mail as an effective teaching supplement. *Educational Technology, 34,* 53–55.

Reinert, B., & Fryback, P. (1997). Distance learning and nursing education. *Journal of Nursing Education, 36,* 421–427.

Ribbons, R. M. (1998). The use of computers as cognitive tools to facilitate higher order thinking skills in nurse education. *Computers in Nursing, 16*(4), 223–227.

Sheridan, M., & LeGros, E. (1995). Computer-assisted instruction using electronic mail. *Journal of Nursing and Staff Development, 11*(2), 100–103.

Sherwood, G. D., Armstrong, M. L., & Bond, M. L. (1994). Distance education programs:Defining issues of assessment, accessibility, and accommodation. *Journal of Continuing Education in Nursing, 25*(8), 251–257.

Shoemaker, D. (1993). A statewide instructional television program via satellite for RN-to-BSN students. *Journal of Professional Nursing, 9*(3), 153–158.

Shutte, J. G. (1997). _Virtual teaching in higher education: The new intellectual superhighway or just another traffic jam?_ [On-line]. Available: http://www.csun.edu/sociology/virexp.htm.

Siktberg, L. L., & Dillard, N. L. (1999). Technology in the nursing classroom. _Nursing and Health Care Perspectives, 20_(3), 128–133.

Skiba, D. (1997). Transforming nursing education to celebrate learning. _Nursing and Healthcare Perspectives, 18_(3), 124–129, 148.

Todd, N. A. (1998). Using E-mail in an undergraduate nursing course to increase critical thinking skills. _Computers in Nursing, 16_(2), 115–118.

Viverais-Dresler, G., & Kutshke, M. (1992). RN students' satisfaction with clinical teaching in a distance education program. _Journal of Continuing Education in Nursing, 23_(5), 224–230.

Wieseke, A., & Pavlechko, G. (1992). A model for open and distance learning for RN baccalaureate nursing students (videocase study). In N. Estes & M. Thomas (Eds.), _The Ninth International Conference on Technology and Education_ (pp. 1063–1065). Austin, TX: The University of Texas at Austin, College of Education.

Wizer, D., & Lynch, W. (1995, April). _The benefits of online education in graduate studies._ Paper presented at AERA Annual Conference, San Francisco.

Wuest, J. (1989). Debate: A strategy for increasing interaction in audio teleconferencing. _Journal of Advanced Nursing, 14,_ 847–852.

Yeaworth, R. C., Benschoter, R. A., Meter, R., & Benson, S. (1995). Telecommunications and nursing education. _Journal of Professional Nursing, 11_(4), 227–232.

7

Promoting Informatics in the Nursing Curriculum

Lucille L. Travis

As the American Association of Colleges of Nursing states in *Nursing Education's Agenda for the 21st Century* (AACN, 1993), nursing education must encompass the requirements for entry into practice and, to the greatest extent possible, anticipate the requirements for nursing practice in the future. With the complex clinical practice of the 21st century, nurses will face escalating information management challenges. Not only will they have to process and communicate more information than ever before, but also the nature and types of information they must handle will change. Information technologies can help nurses meet the challenges but only if nurses can effectively use these technologies. As the use of computer technology and information science increases in nursing practice, education, and administration, so will nurses' need to be skilled and knowledgeable in the use of information technology (Ozbolt, Schultz, Swain, & Abraham, 1985; Ryan, 1985; Saba & McCormick, 1995).

Guidelines for Incorporating Technology into Professional Nursing Education (AACN, 1996) identifies the issue specifically. This encompasses both baccalaureate and higher degree nursing programs. Thus, one challenge facing educators is to develop nurses' abilities to handle a wide range of information technologies. Computerized information systems, electronic monitoring devices, and microprocessor implants are but a few of the computerized devices nurses encounter (Hannah, Ball, & Edwards, 1994; Saba & McCormick, 1995). Besides computerized devices, nursing practice of the future will rely heavily on automated imaging systems, telecomputing, and robotics. We face a challenge not only to make nurses technologically competent but also to produce a new type of graduate who will excel in clinical practice through effective use of information technologies. Both computer literacy and concepts related to nursing informatics should be incorporated into all levels of nursing education. However, computer literacy can be obtained before entering a program or while in the nursing program at various university facilities (Thompson, 1996).

Grier (1981, 1984) has noted the problems that inefficient information handling causes nurses. To avoid incorrect diagnoses, cumbersome assessment strategies, and inappropriate problem identification, it is imperative that nurses recognize from the beginning of their education that, like the basic sciences, information science is a supportive discipline for nursing. Preparing nurses to face the information challenges of the future therefore requires a solid grounding in information sciences; simply teaching computer applications in nursing will not provide nurses with the skills to critically appraise their information needs and evaluate the utility of gathering information in patient care (Hannah et al., 1994; Romano, 1985). This chapter describes a model curriculum in nursing informatics that can be integrated into a 4-year baccalaureate program or adjusted for a master's degree program. All the courses can be taught in a distance format.

Nursing informatics is a combination of "computer science, information science and nursing science designed to assist in the management and processing of nursing data, information and knowledge to support the practice of nursing and the delivery of nursing care" (Graves & Corcoran, 1989, p. 228). An understanding of computers, or computer literacy, is necessary but not sufficient for nursing practice. To ensure that practitioners can meet the challenges that the future holds, it is essential to incorporate the full range of informatics into the education of nurses. Educators must assure that nursing students view the integration of technology into the support of patient care as the appropriate focus of nursing. The disciplines on which informatics courses rest include nursing science, information science, computer technology, and the quantitative foundations of nursing (Graves & Corcoran, 1989; NCNR Priority Expert Panel on Nursing Informatics, 1993; White, 1987).

Argyris and Schon (1974) suggest that clinical field experience in a professional nursing program should not be designed merely to allow students to learn accepted practices but should also provide students with opportunities to try out new approaches and modalities of care. The nursing informatics courses must be designed to articulate with clinical experiences, and the application of information technology must be incorporated into students' clinical experiences. The majority of health care organizations that serve as clinical agencies for nursing students are now using some form of nursing information systems. Therefore, students will have varied opportunities to observe applications in the nursing practice environment.

COURSE DESCRIPTIONS

The model approach to preparing nurses who are competent in informatics is a four-course sequence in which each course develops both conceptual and technical skills. The framework for the informatics curriculum includes information, technology, and clinical care process (Figure 7.1). Each course should address the three components; however, the emphasis on these components will vary with the courses. The courses also must fit with the clinical experience and course progression followed by the students. Supporting coursework in computer science or information science is not required; all the key content is incorporated into the four-course sequence.

The first course in the sequence is Introduction to Nursing Informatics (2 credits). The emphasis is on information and technology, with an overlap in the clinical care process (see Figure 7.1). This course focuses on helping students identify the content, flow, and processing of patient information. In Nursing Informatics II (1 credit), the primary emphasis is on information and the clinical care process, with secondary emphasis on technology (see Figure 7.1). This course prepares the student to handle the quantitative information encountered in the clinical area. In the third course, Nursing Informatics III: Clinical Nursing Information Systems (2 credits), the focus is on the overlap of the three components: information, technology, and clinical care process. The emphasis is on the use of information technologies to support nursing management in clinical applications. The culminating course is Nursing Informatics IV: Applications (2 credits). This course is designed to provide hands-on experience for the student in selected areas of application in nursing informatics (Travis & Brennan, 1998).

Introduction to Nursing Informatics

The prerequisite for the first course is an introduction to computers course. Most students today will have had this introduction in high school or at

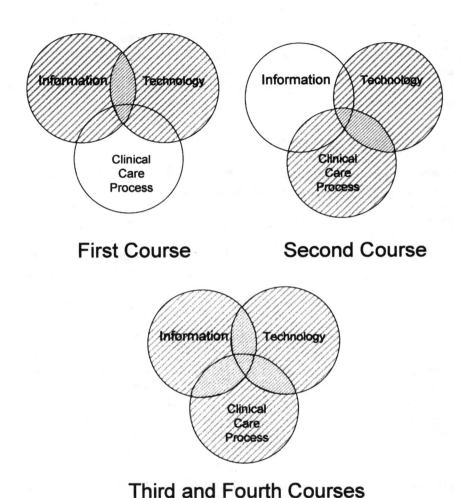

First Course   Second Course

Third and Fourth Courses

FIGURE 7.1   Nursing informatics course framework.

a community college. Students who have not had such an introduction or need an update will have to complete a brief intensive introduction to the computer that is usually offered routinely through a computer support division of a college or university.

The first course in the nursing informatics sequence emphasizes information and technology components, with only a small involvement with the clinical care process because students have had limited clinical experience. The focus is on helping students identify the content, flow, and processing of patient information in the hospital, nursing home, or community agency. It presents the health care organization as an information processor and is based on the premise that the foundation of interdisciplinary communication and decision making is information generated by the patient and through caring for the patient. The information examined is reviewed within the context of the nursing process and the role of the nurse as the gateway for patient information.

The course provides an overview of the key players in the health care environment and the ways in which they influence care delivery. It is also designed to build an understanding of computer technologies and the ways in which nurses can access computers to support them in delivering patient care. The primary objective is to give students a basic understanding of the flow of information through the health care environment and the ways in which information technology can facilitate the collection, processing, and communication of this information. The course should minimally address the following topics: (1) the health care organization as an information processor, (2) the nurse as an information processor, (3) nursing delivery models and information needs, (4) the role of computers in the health care environment, (5) basic data processing theory and terminology, (6) potential of nursing informatics systems, (7) external influences on nursing informatics.

Students can be exposed to knowledge transformation through a series of exercises and lectures. These exercises may utilize the students' beginning knowledge of the Nursing Minimum Data Set or other data in the development of a database specific to an area of practice (e.g., inpatient, community, rehabilitation facility). Additionally, students are given the opportunity to develop a nursing informatics system using instructor-specified parameters and conceptual knowledge.

Nursing Informatics II

The second course should prepare students to handle the information encountered in clinical areas. A computerized hospital simulation program or computerized patient record simulation may be used to help students apply classroom concepts to technology in the health care organization. A broad-based health care computer simulation program presents students with the pieces often lacking in local clinical agency sites. The course focuses on the process of accessing and documenting as well as critically analyzing the computerized patient care record. This hands-on introduction to nursing informatics nurtures an exploration of and appreciation for the computerized patient record. The course also examines the formation, processing, and examination of data and clinical information generated during care delivery.

In this second-level informatics course the electronic patient record is used to expand on the programs' basic documentation functions with the help of instructor-designed assignments, allowing the program to be applied in more creative ways. For example, students can be provided with only the computer data and forced to delegate tasks and make clinical care decisions based on the scenario presented. This reinforces the inherent analytical process in critique of the information-gathering utility of the computerized patient care record.

Exploration of the Minimum Data Set or other data sets can further bring to life the concept of prioritizing the most significant data in order to provide patient care. Within the computerized hospital simulation program, students review incomplete data and learn that some data are more significant than others in planning and delivering the most effective and efficient patient care. This analysis of the "value" of various data sets continues to build critical thinking as the students internalize the concept of a data set.

Second-level students demonstrate their increased knowledge through development and presentation of a project independently determined by a clinical group. The students should be free to utilize any network resources, including computer simulations. Students in the second year also can gain increased understanding of nursing research through use of surveys and resulting data analysis. In addition, this course introduces epidemiologic concepts and biostatistics.

Nursing Informatics III: Clinical Nursing Information Systems

In the third course the focus should be on the intersections of the three components: information, technology, and clinical care process. The emphasis is on the use of information technologies to support nursing management in clinical applications. This course may be offered either in the second semester of the third year or the first semester of the fourth year of a four-year program. The course focuses on giving students an understanding of the relationships between nursing applications and agency-wide computer applications and the impact of nursing interventions on other departments' information processing. Students also develop a thorough understanding of the current and future state of nursing information systems and physiological monitoring systems and their potential for enhancing the nursing process. In addition, they have opportunities to examine the process of planning for, designing, developing, implementing, and evaluating nursing information systems in a clinical environment.

The students also should use application software packages in their clinical courses. Examples of application software include "Nursing Care of Patient with Anxiety Disorder," "Mental Health Simulation, I and II," and "Maternal High Risk—Cardiac," available from MediSim; "Musculoskeletal Assessment," and "Thorax and Lung Assessment," available from Lippincott; and "ABGee," available from Health Sciences Consortium. In addition, examples of interactive videos that students can use include "Nursing Care of the Elderly Cardiac Patient," available from American Journal of Nursing Company; "Concepts and Care of the Immunosuppressed Patient, I and II," available from Health Sciences Consortium; and "IV Therapy," available from Fitne.

The student enters the third level of informatics ready to relate information technology to decision support at the patient, unit, and system levels. Concepts such as management information systems and operational needs are introduced. The benefits of information technology as well as application of system analysis concepts to the decision-making process are included. The process involved in evaluation and selection of a nursing information system are also discussed, as well as the degree of fit between the nursing information system and the nursing care delivery system. Finally, ethical issues related to the use and storage of patient-related data are addressed. In summary, the third course focuses on the outcomes of application and analysis of information technology as related to the patient care process.

Third-level students explore the entire spectrum of informatics technologies available within and outside nursing. Continued emphasis on nursing research and its relationship to informatics gives rise to individual exploration of topics such as virtual reality; the use of a universal, electric medical record; robotics in health care; and the issues of privacy, security, and confidentiality of patient information. The increased flexibility and independence students learn in this course prepare them for the fourth-level informatics course, which emphasizes application of previous informatics knowledge.

Nursing Informatics IV: Applications

The fourth and final course incorporates the knowledge gained in previous courses to build a perspective on the adoption and use of nursing information systems to assist nurses in decision making. It is offered in the final semester of the undergraduate program. This course provides hands-on experience for students in selected areas of application in nursing informatics. The course is project-based: students are grouped into teams of five to seven members to work on agency-specified projects.

The projects that form the core activities of the course originate in health care organizations and meet needs within the agency environment. The relationships of students with clinical agencies help students better understand the nature of information management within the agency and meaningfully participate in informatics projects. To initiate projects, the course instructor should meet with key personnel in each of the participating agencies, including nurse administrators, advanced practice nurses, and information systems coordinators. The concept of nursing informatics projects can be explained as encompassing any work required to enhance nurses' ability to obtain, manage, store, or manipulate the data necessary for practice. Agency personnel should be asked to identify four to six projects per health care organization and to provide the following information for each project: project title, objectives, deliverables, special considerations, and deadlines.

Projects requiring approximately 6 weeks of work (about 200 person-hours) are sought. Projects may include such things as developing a scantron form for recording the critical path of patients with cardiac surgery; constructing a database to help a nurse practitioner–lactation consultant manage her practice; proposing a data access policy for a large university teaching hospital; creating a database to enable staff on a psychiatric inpatient service to conduct follow-up on patients; generating charts and graphs from a mainframe-stored, hours-worked data set; devising a database and screening system to predict patients at risk for discharge planning challenges; establishing the information flow of an outpatient ultrasonography service; providing off-hours backup and training support for a hospital bringing up a new hospital information system, and defining the information requirements necessary to support a continuous quality improvement project.

Projects may vary in the extent of computing skill necessary to conduct the work and the amount of face-to-face interaction required to complete the tasks. Some projects will have no need for computer systems; others, such as database creation activities, will require specific computer skills. All projects should challenge students to work with an agency staff member to define project deliverables, to interact with peers in a task-focused manner, and to apply prior nursing informatics knowledge to solve real-world problems.

Students participate in four class sessions in which the content focuses on team building, project planning, and organizational communication. Students' then self-select into project teams. Under the direction of the course instructor, the student teams spend 6 weeks preparing a project work plan and obtaining the necessary skills and materials to carry out the work plan. Once a project team receives written approval from the course instructor and the agency contact person, the team implements the work plan.

Student teams provide weekly electronic mail updates of project status to the course instructor. Each E-mail message includes the progress toward objectives, accomplishments of the week, and any obstacles to progress, with a plan for managing the obstacles. The course instructor provides weekly feedback. Each project team also maintains a three-ring binder of materials related to the project, including background reading and drafts of work. These binders are kept in a public place accessible to all students.

Students can present the results of their projects to classmates and selected faculty through a variety of methods (e.g., posters with detailed explanation of output presented, demonstration of developed programs on computers, and presentation of deliverables agreed on by the project group).

DEVELOPMENT OF AN INFORMATICS CURRICULUM

In addition to the specific course requirements, other informatics activities should be integrated throughout the curriculum. For example, each student should be required to identify all sources of information obtained and utilized to develop the patient's nursing care plan. Students indicate whether information was obtained through access to the manual chart, the automated computer systems, interviews with patient or family, or inter- and intradepartmental communication. They should indicate the ease or difficulty of collecting and analyzing patient information and also be required to identify opportunities for information technology to enhance the capture, processing, and communication of their own nursing information. This approach not only reinforces the concepts of information capture and communication but also gives the student an opportunity to analyze the voluminous data collected and maintained on patients and to filter that data into clinically relevant information.

In developing an informatics curriculum, it is helpful to enlist the aid of local agency personnel to ensure an integrated perspective. These persons also may participate in teaching the courses, and they will be invaluable in helping students develop meaningful projects in the advanced course.

It is also important to work closely with clinical and other faculty to ensure their support for this approach to informatics and to avoid redundancy in the curriculum. For example, documentation may be covered adequately in the first informatics course and then will not have to be taught in other courses.

Faculty development regarding integration of informatics into the curriculum should be ongoing. For example, assistance with inclusion and expansion of relevant content in the nursing course syllabus will be useful in encouraging faculty involvement. Suggestions regarding course activities will assist faculty in understanding the underlying importance of reinforcing informatics throughout the curriculum.

While this chapter discusses the inclusion of informatics in a baccalaureate nursing program, master's degree programs also should include fundamental informatics components. Faculty must facilitate students' analysis of data elements needed to perform advanced clinical decision and provide accountability for advanced practice activities. Consequently, faculty commitment and expertise is essential to adapt the curriculum for the advanced student.

Distance learning is a strategy that can be incorporated into a variety of courses, particularly the informatics courses. There are numerous mechanisms available to assist faculty in the development of courses for distance format whether through videoconference, videotaping of classes or Internet-based courses. Whether at the undergraduate or graduate level, technical, financial, and pedagogical implications should be assessed and evaluated. Milstead and Nelson (1998) provide a thorough discussion of many common issues faced in using the distance learning strategy.

EVALUATION

Effective evaluation of innovative curricula requires appraisal of three dimensions: course evaluation, student performance, and employer appraisal. One challenge that will be faced by course faculty is stimulating participation by students in courses viewed as not clinical by members of a clinical major. To solve this problem, faculty must communicate the clinical relevance of course assignments in the informatics courses. Another challenge is the disparity between the advanced nursing informatics content presented in the classroom and the lack of sophisticated information technologies for nursing students found in some clinical areas.

Based on the evolving health care environment and technology, new measures must be investigated and employed to effectively evaluate an informatics curriculum. Given the positive results obtained from product outcomes and performance appraisals, it appears that these measures may be useful. Methods that incorporate new and flexible outcome measures will provide opportunities to obtain needed data to evaluate results of curriculum implementation.

The informatics curriculum will have immediate benefits for employers. They will need to spend less time orienting new nurses to the information technology used in the agency, and graduates will quickly be able to apply their general understanding to the specific agency system. When students are exposed to common informatics concepts within the framework of information, technology and the clinical care process, they can become contributing members of the health care team in a relatively short time.

CONCLUSION

The nursing informatics sequence helps students gain the conceptual and psychomotor skills necessary to use information technology effectively in practice. Because we live in a health care environment characterized by technological advances, external pressures, and rapid change, the four-course sequence must continue to evolve to prepare professional nurses to practice in changing environments. Ongoing evaluation by students and faculty will ensure the relevance and timeliness of the curriculum and its contribution to students' future development as professional nurses. The curriculum offers one example of a strategy to achieve the American Association of Colleges of Nursing's (1993) mandate to prepare students for future practice challenges.

REFERENCES

American Association of Colleges of Nursing. (1993). *AACN: Position statement: Nursing education's agenda for the 21st century.* Washington, DC: Author.

American Association of Colleges of Nursing. (1996). *AACN: Guidelines for incorporating technology into professional nursing education.* Washington, DC: Author.

Argyris, C., & Schon, D. (1974). *A theory in practice: Increasing professional effectiveness.* San Francisco: Jossey-Bass.

Graves, J., & Corcoran, S. (1989). The study of nursing informatics. *Image, 21*(4), 227–231.

Grier, M. (1981). On the need for data in making nursing decisions. In H. Werley & M. Grier (Eds.), *Nursing information systems* (pp. 15–31). New York: Springer Publishing Co.

Grier, M. (1984). Information processing in nursing. In H. Werley & J. Fitzpatrick (Eds.), *Annual review of nursing research* (pp. 265–287). Philadelphia: W. B. Saunders.

Hannah, K. J., Ball, M. J., & Edwards, M. J. (1994). *Introduction to nursing informatics.* New York: Springer-Verlag.

Milstead, J. A., & Nelson, R. (1998). Preparation for an online asynchronous university doctoral course: Lessons learned. *Computers in Nursing, 16*(5), 247–258.

National Center for Nursing Research, Priority Expert Panel on Nursing Informatics. (1993). *Nursing informatics: Enhancing patient care.* Bethesda, MD: National Center for Nursing Research, National Institutes of Health, Public Health Service, U.S. Department of Health and Human Services.

Ozbolt, J. G., Schultz, S., II, Swain, M. A., & Abraham, I. L. (1985). A proposed expert system for nursing practice: A springboard to nursing science. *Journal of Medical Systems, 9*(1–2), 57–68.

Romano, C. A. (1985). Computer technology and nursing: A futuristic view. *Computers in Nursing, 3*(2), 85–87.

Ryan, S. A. (1985). An expert system for nursing practice: Clinical decision support. *Computers in Nursing, 3*(2), 77–84.

Saba, V. K., & McCormick, K. A. (1995). *Essentials of computers for nurses.* New York: McGraw-Hill.

Thompson, C. B. (1996). Infomatics and computer literacy: In master's education via interdisciplinary links, case management, and nursing informatics. *Proceedings of the American Association of Colleges of Nursing's Master's Education Conference.* Washington, DC: AACN.

Travis, L. L., & Brennan, P. (1998). Information science for the future: An innovative nursing informatics curriculum. *Journal of Nursing Education, 37*(4), 162–168.

White, M. (Ed.). (1987). *What curriculum for the information age.* Hillsdale, NJ: Erlbaum.

8

Distance Education at the University of Phoenix

JoAnn Zerwekh and Sandra W. Pepicello

The University of Phoenix (UOP) is America's largest private, accredited university for working adults, with over 61,000 enrolled students. First accredited in 1978, UOP has maintained an ability to understand and meet the needs of the working adult student. By responding to the need of this type of student, UOP has remodeled the boundaries of the classroom and, in the case of on-line education and directed study, has eliminated the classroom altogether.

In nearly two decades of developing and implementing targeted academic programs, UOP has achieved an enviable ability to understand and meet the specialized demands of the working student. Today, UOP offers a multitude of programs at learning center locations across 81 campuses in 14 states, the Commonwealth of Puerto Rico, and Vancouver, British Columbia, and via on-line distance education. The university is accredited by the Commission on Institutions of Higher Education of the North Central Association of Colleges and Schools (NCA).

The cornerstone of UOP's educational philosophy is recognition of the distinction between the younger student still deciding on a career and the adult student who has established personal and professional goals, and offers working adults a program that assists them to integrate their full personal and professional lives by allowing the important benefit that occurs from the integration of work and school. With over 6,200 faculty members, composed of part-time working practitioners who are experts in their field, UOP excels in providing up-to-date, real-world experience for its students. This committed cadre of faculty, who have advanced academic preparation and professional experience, participate in the college-wide faculty governance system.

MISSION STATEMENT

The University of Phoenix is a private, for-profit higher education institution whose mission is to provide high-quality education to working adult students. The university identifies educational needs and provides, through innovative methods (including distance education technologies), educational access to working adults regardless of their geographical location. The university provides general education and professional programs that prepare students to articulate and advance their personal and professional goals.

The university's educational philosophy and operational structure embody participative, collaborative, and applied problem-solving strategies that are facilitated by a faculty whose advanced academic preparation and professional experience help integrate academic theory with current practical application. The university assesses both the effectiveness of its academic offerings and the academic achievement of its students and utilizes the results of these assessments to improve academic and institutional quality.

FACULTY GOVERNANCE STRUCTURE

Academic governance at the university reflects the unique characteristics of the institution, its mission, and its practicing faculty. The governance structure is designed to maximize participation by faculty and to assure that faculty members are able to communicate effectively with each other as well as with the university administration. The core of the university governance structure is the Academic Cabinet, which includes, as voting members, senior administrators, the university deans, and practitioner faculty representing each of the university's main campus locations. The Academic Cabinet has responsibility for approving programs, curriculum, and academic policies and for affirming actions taken by the university's colleges through their respective central curriculum committees. Faculty representatives to the cabinet are chosen at each campus from among the group of highly qualified practitioner faculty who serve as assistant department chairs for the various colleges. The full-time faculty members of the university are campus department chairs, located at each campus and required to teach, review, and revise curriculum and participate in academic governance as well as maintain oversight of the college's programs (University of Phoenix (1999). Online Campus. [On-line]. Available: http://www.online.uophx.edu.).

COLLEGE OF NURSING AND HEALTH SCIENCES

The College of Nursing and Health Sciences was established to respond to the educational needs of registered nurses. The college offers working nurses opportunities to participate in degree programs developed to broaden their professional horizons. These programs are designed specifically for nurses who desire a repertoire of skills and knowledge necessary to respond effectively to today's dynamic health care environment. They also equip nurses with essential skills necessary to assume a leadership role in resolving the challenges being faced by health care organizations and personnel. Each program has a blend of theory and practice, fostering a learning environment that allows nurses to build their knowledge base and to apply, effectively and creatively, what they have learned. The college currently offers the following National League for Nursing Accrediting Commission (NLNAC) accredited degree programs:

- Bachelor of Science in Nursing (BSN)
- Master of Science in Nursing (MSN)
- Master of Science in Nursing/Women's Health Care Nurse Practitioner[*]
- Master Science Nursing/Family Nurse Practitioner[*]

[*]Programs that can be taken at selected UOP campuses.

Campus or Ground-based Courses

The College of Nursing and Health Sciences has been able to develop innovative yet convenient programs. By taking one course at a time, one night a week in a classroom setting, students are able to focus on learning and skill building, which is preferred by working students. Additionally, the school's programs promote team-building competencies through weekly study group meetings needed to complete course outcomes. The program runs through the calendar year, allowing students to start at their convenience. This ground-based delivery of the nursing programs serves 90% of the university's nursing student body.

Students are registered for their entire academic program at one time. Tuition is then paid at the first class of each course, and course materials, including texts and readings, can be delivered in advance. All students are provided library services through the university's extensive Online Learning Resource Center.

Directed Study: The One-on-One Format

In addition to the ground-based delivery format, the nursing programs also are offered through distance education modalities serving 10% of the university's nursing student body. Even though the delivery of content and the student/teacher interaction is varied, students must achieve the same outcomes as do students who are in the more traditional classroom environment. Some modification is necessary for the completion of assignments. For example, classroom students are required to develop oral communication skills by conducting presentations in front of their classmates. Distance education students develop these same skills by conducting oral presentations on audio- or videocassette to be evaluated by the faculty.

Most of the on-line degree programs utilize a group-based format, where small groups of students interact via E-mail forums. However, because a few programs require more individualized instruction, they are offered in a one-to-one format. These programs include bachelor of science in nursing, master of science in nursing, and master of arts in education.

In these programs the student is matched with a faculty member for each class, who guides them through course material on a one-to-one basis. Via E-mail the instructor evaluates the student's work, offers feedback, and provides encouragement on a weekly basis. Students are encouraged to ask frequent questions and engage in dialogue with their instructor. Written assignments are due at the end of each week and are returned to the student in 48 hours with instructor comments, feedback, and grades. Students have the opportunity to work with faculty who are nursing experts and live in locations all across the country.

On-line: The Group-based Format

The on-line delivery modality at the university was formed in 1989 and currently has an enrollment of 9,800 degree-seeking adult students from all over the United States and the world (A. Collins, personal communication, August 11, 1999). It is a group-based learning environment offering the kind of interaction and support that takes place in a traditional face-to-face seminar-style classroom. The University of Phoenix Online offers unparalleled convenience and flexibility of attending classes from a personal computer. In small groups of 8 to 13 or working one-to-one with an instructor, students discuss issues, share ideas, and test theories.

On-line computer-mediated education was an outgrowth of the technological transformation of the workplace and a response to the increasing use of computers and modems for communication. Since 1989, UOP's computer-based educational delivery system has extended the boundaries of the classroom. The on-line program uses the power of the Internet to deliver on-line learning that is independent of time and location. Rather than gathering in a classroom, students and instructors interact on-line or off-line in a forum using Microsoft® technology (see Figure 8.1).

In the on-line program, communication is many-to-many rather than one-to-one. Each class shares its own group mailbox, which serves as an "electronic classroom." Although communication between individuals is common, each class uses a group forum where students put their work and ideas before classmates for comment. This upgrades the quality of most work before its more formal, academic review by the instructor.

The on-line program is designed to benefit working professionals in a number of ways. Classes are offered one at a time, in sequence. There are no semesters, so students can begin a course of study any month of the year. A student can concentrate on one subject at a time, and when a class is completed, he or she can move on to the next one until all degree requirements are met.

Each on-line class lasts 5 or 6 weeks. A student can sign on any hour of the day or night, taking part at times that best fit his or her schedule.

Recommended Hardware

(Microsoft® Windows 95/98)
Pentium 75 or better with 32MB RAM or more
1GB HD or better, CD-ROM
SVGA monitor, 28.8 baud or faster modem, Internet access
Windows-based word processing and spreadsheet applications are required for on-line programs.
The MBA/TM program requires project management software in addition to word processing and spreadsheet applications.

While this flexibility is unprecedented, it requires greater than average discipline and does not allow a student to "coast." Students devote an average of 15 to 20 hours a week to their studies.

On-line Faculty

Although proficient in their fields, on-line faculty members must also go through extensive on-line training to prepare them to teach effectively in an on-line environment. The training begins with a self-paced technical tutorial and proficiency exam, then continues with a comprehensive training course conducted entirely on-line. Finally, all faculty are mentored in their first classes with the aid of both process and content experts; they must meet rigorous standards for both content knowledge and facilitation skills to pass the mentorship portion of the selection process.

Although prospective instructors are focused on the initial training and mentorship processes at UOP, on-line faculty training literally never stops. Additional development courses enhance instructional skills and keep them up to date. Workshop topics include on-line communication techniques, grading and assessment, and adult learning theories, to name just a few. Continuing education sessions, as well as faculty meetings to discuss and inform on-line curriculum development, are conducted entirely on-line.

What an On-line Course Is Like

Typically, on the first day of the week the instructor sends introductory information on the week's topic and confirms the assignments, such as reading from the textbook, completing a case study, or preparing a paper on the topic identified in the module.

The instructor also posts a short lecture or elaborates on the material and provides discussion questions related to the topic. Throughout the week the student works on reading and assignments, just as in a traditional classroom setting. The student uses the computer conferencing system to participate in the class discussion, asks questions, and receives feedback. When assignments are due, the student sends them to the instructor on-line, she or he grades them, and sends them back to the student with comments.

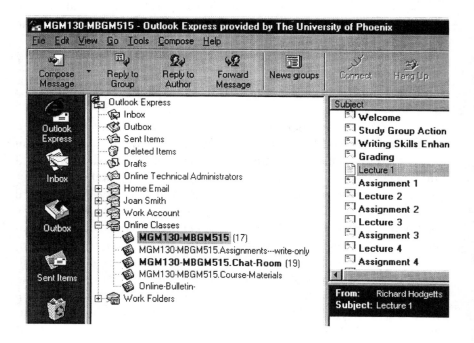

FIGURE 8.1   Microsoft® Outlook Express.

THE NURSING PROGRAMS

MSN Programs

The MSN programs are developed for nurses who want to ground their professional nursing decisions and actions with appropriate nursing theories, research principles, and practices. The MSN curricula build on baccalaureate education through the development of advanced practice roles of caregiver, teacher, and manager of care.

The MSN programs are designed to develop and enhance the knowledge and skills of registered nurses. They are also designed for those nurses who want to pursue more advanced positions in today's challenging health care environment. The programs blend nursing theory with advanced practice concepts necessary to work successfully within the structure, culture, and mission of any-size health care organization or educational setting.

The MSN programs consist of three major areas: the core, the major, and the cognate. The core incorporates the major foci of a master of nursing degree: the theory of nursing, ethical nursing issues, and the influence of nursing research on the advanced practice of nursing. The major, depending on student choice, includes either advanced course work in nursing management of families and aggregates, administration, and education or course work directed toward nurse practitioner focus. The cognate that occurs in the aggregate-based MSN includes course work concerning today's health care environment: health care infrastructure, health care finance, and data-based decision making. Classes meet in formal session once each week for 4 hours. Additional time is required outside class for homework, study group meetings, and project activities.

Table 8.1 lists the course of study for the MSN program that does not include the nurse practitioner component.

Bachelor of Science in Nursing

The bachelor of science in nursing (BSN) program is built on a foundation of biological, physical, and social sciences that contribute to the science of nursing. The liberal arts components enhance the development of the

TABLE 8.1   MSN Course of Study

Course No.	Course Title
HCS 501	Introduction to Nursing Graduate Studies (2 credits)
NUR 515.3	Advanced Nursing Theory (3 credits)
NUR 540	Advanced Nursing Management: Individuals and Families (3 credits)
NUR 543	Advanced Nursing Management: Communities (3 credits)
HCS 520	Health Care Infrastructure (3 credits)
HCS 583	Data Based Decision Making (3 credits)
NUR 576	Ethical Issues in Nursing (2 credits)
HCS 581.3	Change, Negotiation, and Conflict Resolution in Health Care (3 credits)
NUR 597AO	Nursing Research Project Orientation (0 credits)
NUR 584	Dynamics of Nursing Administration (3 credits)
HCS 582	Health Care Finance (3 credits)
NUR 586.3	Curriculum Development and Program Design (3 credits)
NUR 597A	Nursing Research Project (3 credits)
NUR 597B	Nursing Research Project (2 credits)
NUR 590A	Nursing Practicum (1 credit)
NUR 590B	Nursing Practicum (2 credits)

intellectual, social, and cultural aspects of the professional nurse. One hallmark of the BSN program is that there is no testing of prior knowledge if the RN is a graduate of an NLNAC or regionally accredited program. The BSN program is designed to develop the professional knowledge and skills of working registered nurses without the need to relearn nursing content already acquired in prior academic programs.

The program enhances the foundation in the biological, physical, and social sciences through an instructional program with behavioral objectives that concentrate on the development of the nurse's role as caregiver, teacher, and manager of care. Utilizing a self-care framework, working registered nurses are prepared as generalists who are able to apply professional skills and knowledge to nursing, client, and health care systems.

Table 8.2 outlines the BSN required course of study.

BSN/MSN Program Pathway

Students planning to continue on to the master of science nursing program may complete up to nine graduate credits as part of their upper-division

TABLE 8.2   BSN Course of Study

Course No.	Course Title
Nursing core courses	
NUR 401	Theoretical Foundations for Professional Nursing (4 credits)
NUR 417	Pathophysiology and Health Assessment I (3 credits)
NUR 418	Pathophysiology and Health Assessment II (3 credits)
NUR 452	Health Law and Ethics (4 credits)
NUR 464	Concepts of Family Nursing Theory (3 credits)
NUR 465	Clinical Integration: Nursing Management of Families (5 credits)
NUR 429	Issues and Strategies in Nursing Research Utilization (3 credits)
NUR 471	Dimensions of Community Nursing Practice (3 credits)
NUR 472	Clinical Integration Partnerships in Community Practice (4 credits)
NUR 485	Nursing Leadership and Management in Health Care (4 credits)
Cognate courses	
HCS 418	Skills for Professional Transition (3 credits)
HCS 408	Therapeutic Health Care Communications (3 credits)
GEN 323	Professional Ethics and Social Responsibility (3 credits)
QNT 436	Statistics in Health Care (3 credits)

nonnursing elective credit requirements. These courses may be taken only after completing the required course of study.

Sigma Theta Tau

Sigma Theta Tau is an international nursing honor society and a member of the Association of College Honor Societies. Chartered in 1998, the UOP chapter's purposes are to foster high professional standards, to encourage creative work, to promote the maximum development of the individual, and to strengthen commitment to the ideals and purposes of the profession of nursing. Invitation to membership is extended to students and other members of the nursing community who have demonstrated qualities of leadership and capacity for professional growth. Students are notified of membership eligibility annually, based on grade point average.

CONCLUSION

With over 3,000 nursing students on 20 campuses and over 1,000 clinical placements, UOP's nursing program is one of the largest in the country. The university is committed to excellence in nursing education in an innovative, model delivery format of ground-based, directed study and on-line education that provides up-to-date, real-world experience for its students. The University of Phoenix strives to be the exemplar of adult education in the next millennium, or in the words of President Jorge Klor de Alva (1999), "The future is here!"

REFERENCES

Collins, A. (1999). (Personal communication), August 11, 1999.
Klor de Alva, J. (1999, July). Address to University of Phoenix faculty at annual retreat, Phoenix, AZ. (1999). University of Phoenix. Online Campus [Online]. Available: http://www.online.uophx.edu.

9

Distance Graduate Education: The University of Colorado Experience

Joan K. Magilvy and Marlaine C. Smith

We are in the midst of a technological revolution that is changing the face of graduate education in nursing. Master's degree education in nursing is designed to prepare nurses for advanced practice roles and entry into doctoral programs, whereas doctoral education is designed to prepare nurse scientists and innovators, those contributing to the knowledge of the discipline. Outreach programs in graduate education have been developed to increase access, but few have developed totally off-site opportunities for students. Students have had to travel for a portion of their learning experiences to the campus, for classroom or clinical instruction. With burgeoning access to technology that can support quality remote teaching-learning, greater numbers of nurses will have access to master's and doctoral degrees as well as bundled curriculum modules that can help them develop career competencies.

With the strong emphasis on technology and information management in health care and health professional education, graduate programs in nursing must facilitate the development of flexible, knowledgeable, and technologically competent practitioners, researchers, administrators, and leaders. Technology has "dramatically altered practice, teaching, and learning environments in nursing as well as the way in which nurses, educators, and students communicate" (American Association of Colleges of Nursing [AACN], 1997, p. 6). The AACN recommends that to improve teaching methods at all program levels, advanced technology and creative learning approaches should be incorporated into nursing curricula.

Within this context of a holistic learning environment, all possible teaching and learning strategies and modes of delivery of instruction are considered, putting faculty and students into partnership to develop knowledge and engage in scholarship (Siktberg & Dillard, 1999; Skiba, 1997). Mark Schroeder, a former professor turned software-training entrepreneur, commented that, although perceived by many as revolutionary, on-line learning is "a natural evolution of education from Socratic dialogue to written text, to digital technology, [and] is merely an extension of our capabilities, a way to expand our ability to learn" (Appleborne, 1999, p. 37).

The University of Colorado has embarked on a Total Learning Environment Campaign, with several themes, including supporting innovations in learning; responding to students and other constituents; and using technology to improve teaching, learning, research, and management (press release, University of Colorado, October 10, 1996). The university is committed to stimulate development of accessible and expansive educational strategies and technologies, a goal shared by all four campuses. Congruent with a total learning environment, the University of Colorado Health Sciences Center (UCHSC) School of Nursing (SON) has made a strong commitment to making its programs and classes accessible to citizens of Colorado as well as nationally and internationally, using a variety of teaching-learning strategies and technologies.

Since the late 1970s the SON has been engaged in distance learning for graduate education. Diverse methods have been used to deliver programs and courses first to students residing across rural Colorado in the early years, then to students residing across the United States and Canada, and now to nurses worldwide who desire career and educational advancement. Early delivery strategies ranged from faculty driving or flying to rural sites to hold classes on weekends to students who drove from 1 to 4 hours to the teaching site. The summer-only option in the doctoral program was the school's attempt to provide greater access to doctoral education for national and international students who could study in Colorado for 4 summers to complete their PhD coursework. Today, the UCHSC SON delivers courses in interactive video format, on-line and Internet platforms or on-campus in traditional weekly classes, intensive classes of 1–2 weeks, and courses using a combination of these strategies. In addition to traditional classroom seminars and lectures, instructional resources include interactive video with capability of computer, videotape, photographic slide or transparency audiovisuals; Web-based software offering an on-line seminar format with primarily asynchronous discussions, synchronous discussions, and chat rooms; faculty or student-developed presentations; and computer video cameras.

As we are carried away in the throes of this technological revolution, it is essential that we don't toss out the "baby with the bath water." Technology-assisted education is not a frivolous bandwagon. It is here to stay. And while we develop our graduate programs to integrate technology, we must do so reflectively, blending the best of the old with the promises of the new. The purpose of this chapter is to share our reflections and experiences of developing MS and PhD curricula for delivery to rural, national, and international student populations. We will provide some perspectives of changes in graduate education and, as an exemplar, a history of the SON's distance initiatives in graduate education. The strengths and challenges identified by students and faculty during course and program evaluation and suggestions for approaches and solutions will be discussed.

CHANGING CONTEXTS

Consistent with the explosive changes in health care delivery, graduate nursing education has an obligation to act rather than react and shape practice and education rather than respond to a changing environment—in essence, to be the agents of change (AACN, 1997). In a recent position statement on the future of nursing education, the AACN states that, among other mandates, nursing education is responsible for preparing nurses to hold full partnership in health care delivery, shaping health policy, and shaping the health care environment. Particularly, master's education programs will prepare advanced practice nurses for the rapidly changing practice arena, including nurses in indirect care roles of management, administration, and informatics who will be leaders in health care delivery. Doctoral programs in nursing, in addition to developing clinically relevant research and knowledge, have a mandate to prepare future faculty that will engage in new models of education (AACN, 1997). By advancing teaching and learning strategies and using emerging technology, faculty can provide opportunities for students to participate in technology-assisted education, practice, and research. Faculty will model exemplary teaching, promoting in graduates a readiness to be leaders and innovators in the discipline.

With the strong emphasis on technology and information management in health care and health professional education, graduate programs in nursing must facilitate the development of flexible, knowledgeable, and technologically competent practitioners, researchers, administrators, and leaders. Technology has "dramatically altered practice, teaching and learning environments in nursing as well as the way in which nurses, educators, and students communicate" (AACN, 1997, p. 6). The AACN recommends that to improve teaching methods at all program levels, advanced technology and creative learning approaches are needed.

In this time of transformational change, traditional ideologies and methods are supplanted by emergent ones that radically alter the face of our institutions. Table 9.1 shows the paradigms of traditional and emergent perspectives of graduate education in nursing. In the traditional view of

TABLE 9.1 Traditional and Emergent Paradigms of Education

Traditional Paradigm	Emergent Paradigm
Teacher-centered	Learner-centered
Teacher is repository and dispenser of knowledge.	Teacher is guide, coach, facilitator, and designer of learning experiences.
Learner is passive; teacher is responsible.	Learner is active and responsible.
Content and process-focused	Outcomes or competency-focused
Teacher is the arbiter and gatekeeper of knowledge.	Learner negotiates multiple information systems.
Co-facilitation of learning by self-selected clusters.	Co-facilitation of learning by community of learners.
On site learning vs. outreach	All students may be remote learners.
Learning is time- and space-bound.	Learning is anytime and anywhere.
Technology is supportive.	Technology is central.
Face-to-face mentoring, strong with relationships	Asynchronous and nonlocal mentoring, with strong relationships
"Received authority"	"Constructed knowledge"
Incremental learning toward degrees, prescribed and rigid curriculum.	Lifelong learning, ease in access and articulation, bundled units for competencies
Separation of disciplines and departments in educational enterprise	Interdisciplinary partnerships
Practice learning exclusively through on-site clinical placements	Practice learning through simulations, cases, CDs, virtual reality
Academic use of practice sites/settings	Community-campus partnerships
Separation of academicians and practitioners	Expanded network of practice experts involved in teaching and evaluating

graduate education the learner seeks the expertise of the faculty and often selects a graduate program in order to study with selected faculty. The learner studies "at the feet" of the faculty sage, considered the repository of the knowledge necessary for expertise in the field. Knowledge, then, reflects "received authority." Faculty serve as lecturers or seminar leaders and are expected to provide the most current perspectives on the content in the field. In this paradigm faculty are responsible for the development of curriculum, delivery of content, and evaluation of students' knowledge and expertise. While the graduate student is fully engaged in independent learning activities, she or he still may be relatively passive in the identification and structuring of those activities. Certainly, communities of learners grow as graduate students gather to discuss or study together; however, acknowledgment of the value of this process is not routinely structured into learning activities. Mentoring is a hallmark of graduate education. Faculty mentoring of students occurs during intensive face-to-face encounters through shared work and dialogue.

Some graduate programs have attempted to become more accessible through outreach education to rural sites or through developing intensive learning experiences on site, such as summer doctoral education. In these models, students are often viewed as different from the traditional on-site students. In some schools, graduate students are admitted to "departments" that govern admission and graduation standards. The autonomy of these departments leads to limited opportunities for interdisciplinary education, other than a few credits of electives or cognates. In advanced practice education, students often dichotomize the theoretical knowledge taught in the classroom by academics from the practicums precepted by expert clinicians or practitioners. In many cases very little dialogue exists between these two worlds.

The emergent paradigm reflects significant differences that affect graduate education. First, although graduate education is more learner-centered than at the undergraduate level, this quality is even more pronounced. The graduate educator in the new paradigm performs in the role of a guide, coach, facilitator, and architect of the learning experience. The learner is more responsible for building, seeking, and synthesizing appropriate knowledge and experiences. With the recognition that knowledge is growing and changing exponentially, the emphasis on content knowledge is replaced by the focus on outcomes or competence, such as lifelong learning that includes access and negotiation of information systems. Learning becomes asynchronous and nonlocal; that is, it occurs when it is appropriate and convenient for the learner. Communities are structured to facilitate learning through discussion, feedback, and group work. These communities are as central to learning as the teacher.

Graduate education in the new paradigm reflects the need to acquire specified knowledge that is part of an individual's life learning plan. There is greater ease in articulating across departments, disciplines, and programs to seek these competencies. For graduate nursing education, greater opportunity for simulated learning exists through CD-ROMs, Web-based resources, and virtual reality simulations. This paradigm features academic-practitioner partnerships in faculty practices and greater appreciation of practice experts in teaching and evaluating competence.

HISTORICAL PERSPECTIVE

In this context, the UCHSC graduate programs in nursing have moved to an environment of emerging teaching-learning strategies and technologies. As the flagship state higher education institution, a research-intensive setting, and the only health sciences center and doctoral nursing education program in Colorado, the UCHSC has honored a strong commitment to provision of graduate education statewide. Colorado is a predominantly rural state with one major metropolitan area and several smaller cities located along the eastern slope of the Rocky Mountains. Nurses living in the four original Area Health Education Center (AHEC) regions have requested accessible graduate nursing education programs to assist them in advancing their own practice and improving health care delivery to rural Coloradans. Although unable to leave their positions and families to travel to Denver for their graduate studies, these nurses have continually made strong commitments to undertaking master's degree and, more recently, doctoral education. The UCHSC SON has delivered distance education through a variety of strategies for the past 20 years.

On-site

One strategy for delivering education to distant students is on-site education. An extended campus can be accomplished through delivery at remote sites or through intensive delivery at the campus site. Both have been part of the SON's history with increasing access to graduate education.

Since the late 1970s, faculty at the SON traveled to students to offer education throughout rural Colorado. Clusters or cohorts of students were identified at various locations. These cohorts decided on an advanced practice area of study and the courses for that program option were taught by faculty who traveled to remote sites. Students sacrificed their weekends to attend classes. Many in very rural locations traveled as long as 4 hours to arrive at the designated on-site location in Grand Junction, Durango, LaJunta, and elsewhere. This model was used by about eight cohorts of master's degree students studying community health, nursing administration, and primary care. Both faculty and students committed time and energy to travel and engage in the teaching-learning process. They communicated by telephone or, more recently, E-mail during interim periods between classes. The library and bookstore offered distance support services to the students; services included mailing books and articles, interlibrary loans, faxing, and telephone referencing assistance. However, accessing resources for graduate-level work is still an issue for many students.

Another model of on-site instruction is the intensive format. Used by many universities, this format was adopted for our doctoral program to increase access to students working full-time in academic years, in clinical settings or rural sites. Students travel to campus for an intensive course, usually scheduled on consecutive days for 1 week to 2 months. In the late 1980s the UCHSC SON developed a summer-only option in the PhD program to provide access to students in academic or clinical roles who were not free to enroll in year-round full-time study.

Students traveled to Colorado for courses and maintained contact with faculty via telephone until E-mail provided an alternative way to communicate. Courses were delivered in a summerlong intensive format that was extremely demanding of students and faculty alike. Without an opportunity to synthesize and integrate new knowledge, learning was fragmented; faculty recently decided to close this option and develop an option more conducive to year-round learning. The intensive format will be used in the newly developed model expanding the PhD program to international students who will either travel to Colorado for these courses or engage in intensive study in their home region taught by traveling UCHSC faculty. The new model will employ a combination of teaching-learning strategies, including on-site and online courses.

On-screen

In the mid-1990s, facilitated by several grants, the SON and the UCHSC campus built its technology infrastructure and connected the UCHSC with all AHEC offices and several community colleges or smaller state colleges. This technology allowed interactive video classes to be broadcast to as many as eight sites, even to several simultaneously, although many classes were sent to only one or two sites at a time. Two interactive video classrooms were constructed in the SON and School of Medicine. One large classroom seats 30 students on-site and has television monitors that broadcast communications from students in remote sites.

The on-campus and remote sites have technicians that act as educational producers through operating cameras, maintaining the open transmission lines, recording the classes, facilitating effective use of equipment, and communicating with remote-site technicians. With this assistance, faculty can concentrate on teaching. Fax, telephone, computer-assisted presentations, slides, and videos enhance the effectiveness of learning through this medium. The compressed video has about a 3-second delay in transmission. Students at both locations learn to use microphones when they speak in the classroom. With practice, both students and faculty forget the technology and develop creative and entertaining teaching methods to make the classes enjoyable and interesting. A valuable by-product is that students across the state are able to meet and learn with each other.

On-line

In the late 1990s fully on-line courses were initiated although two previous courses used E-mail and distribution lists to facilitate on-line seminar conferencing. The Office of Informatics in the SON supports the development of courses and use of WebCT software. This office collaborates with the Academic Affairs office in faculty development, course evaluation, and grant-writing to support further development of online education.

A regional initiative propelled the growth of distance education at the SON. The Mountain and Plains Partnership (MAPP) Project was developed under the Robert Wood Johnson Foundation Partnerships for Training Initiative. The purpose of the project is to plan and implement distance learning strategies that provide interdisciplinary didactic curricula to community-based health care providers/residents pursuing health-professional education leading to an advanced practice degree and/or certification as a primary care midlevel clinician (physician assistant, nurse practitioner, or certified nurse midwife). MAPP is a collaborative project involving eight educational partners in Colorado and Wyoming. Rural students serving medically underserved communities are able to stay in their communities while pursuing their education as primary care providers. The faculty consortium has developed on-line core courses that can be accessed by MAPP students. Each student receives a computer and computer training for accessing the on-line instruction.

The majority of courses are offered in an *asynchronous* manner (interactive, but delays occur between sending and receiving communication, as in E-mail); however, some faculty have used *synchronous* (immediate communication as in face-to-face, or "live," communication) teaching methods when appropriate. Currently, 15 courses in the master's degree program and 9 courses in the doctoral program are taught on-line.

With this historical and environmental context for technology-supported and distance education, the UCHSC SON continues to develop strategies to facilitate student learning and remote access. Although the PhD program is not planning a fully on-line delivery as Duquesne University in Pittsburgh recently implemented (Milstead & Nelson, 1998), plans are underway to deliver the program with a combination of intensive on-campus classes, traditional courses, and on-line education targeted to a national and international student population. All students in the year-round traditional academic program and the alternative model offering will be free to take courses in any format offered.

The master's program currently offers courses in a variety of on-line, classroom, interactive video, and clinical formats. All 14 credits of core courses are now offered in an on-line as well as a classroom format. Courses in pathophysiology, drug management, health promotion and wellness, advanced assessment, case management, and specialty courses in the primary care of families and oncology nursing options have been offered by Internet or interactive video. Future plans for the master's program include capability to deliver curricula of about five of our MS options totally on-line with remote clinical practica and competency evaluations. This will be delivered via a joint venture with a national educational cable and on-line company and developing strategies for clinical placement and competency evaluation. To support these multiple models of graduate education and make them accessible to students in urban and rural Colorado, across the United States and Canada, and to nurses worldwide, a strong infrastructure and support services are required.

STRENGTHS AND CHALLENGES

Both faculty and students identified numerous strengths and challenges related to distance learning, especially interactive video and on-line courses. Evaluations provide opportunities to examine problems and develop immediate solutions facilitating satisfaction and retention of students. Student perspectives followed by perceptions of faculty will be discussed.

Student Perspectives of Strengths

Students identified strengths of distance education, including flexibility, access, cost savings, diversity of classmates, equalizing cultural and social barriers, currency of discussions, and computer competency. In on-line courses, students commented in evaluations that they appreciated the *flexibility* of participating in on-line discussion at times convenient to their schedules. Many of our students practice or teach, and without compromising their work schedules they are able to complete assignments and participate in seminar discussions in varying blocks of time. They are able to travel for work or vacations as long as they have access to a computer and the Internet.

Both on-line and on-screen interactive video courses were considered to be very *accessible* to remote students. Many of our rural students reported that without this technology they would have been unable to earn a graduate degree as they are place-bound, and staffing shortages preclude taking extended educational leaves. International students, especially in developing countries, may be able to gather sufficient resources to travel for intensive courses or engage in on-line courses from their home countries. Many of these students would be unable to obtain support for full-time on-site study in the United States.

Students evaluated *cost-savings* aspects of distance education as a high priority. Learning from home or in their local area meant that students incurred fewer child care, parking, and auto expenses. With asynchronous learning, use of vacation days for educational purposes was unnecessary.

International PhD students engaged in full-time study had to relocate for 4 to 5 years at considerable expense; the opportunity to engage in intermittent intensive and on-line courses will be very cost-effective in economically challenging times.

Distance education affords graduate students an opportunity to study with a *diverse group* of classmates. Rural and urban, domestic and international, culturally and ethnically diverse students learn together in a virtual classroom, maximizing cross-cultural understanding. *Sociocultural inequalities* are minimized through on-line discussion. Class discussions are more balanced between shy and extroverted students; students of cultural backgrounds that emphasize noncompetitiveness or deference to authority are more likely to participate in an on-line environment. For example, we have observed that international students who never speak in the classroom share critical reflections and cultural experiences in on-line seminars.

Currency of discussion is facilitated by the on-line course format. Discussions take place in a series of course-related forums, each of which can allow for asynchronous and intermittent dialogue by students and faculty. Students can easily search the Web for current resources and bring pertinent new information to seminar discussions immediately. Community events or media stories can be woven into discussion in the various forums. For example, during a doctoral course on the environmental context of health and health care delivery a tragic school shooting occurred, with 15 deaths. Students welcomed the opportunity to discuss the tragedy and its meaning and also critically analyzed social, political, cultural, and community environmental implications; weighed possible interventions; and identified potential research ideas. In the traditional classroom, discussion of this topic might have occurred for one or two class periods, but in an on-line format the discussion could be revisited and explored continuously from multiple perspectives in a separate forum for that purpose while other course topical discussions continued uninterrupted.

Finally, students commented on their increased confidence and *competency* in the use of technology. Interactive video students learned to use computer-assisted presentations and became proficient in the use of many other aspects of instructional technology. On-line students commented on the variety of learning strategies integrated into their courses. Students enjoyed the fact that online courses were modeled after the seminar format used in other master's and doctoral courses. The doctoral students especially recommended that a more didactic or structured approach not be used in on-line instruction. They developed skill in on-line presentations, sharing of reaction papers, debates, leadership of seminars with introductions, discussion questions, monitored dialogues, and formal summarization, and ongoing discussion of current events related to course content. A greater number of master's degree students were computer novices at the beginning of their on-line instruction but rapidly developed competence in computer literacy. This outcome was valued by students and was an important outcome of this learning modality.

Student Challenges

In addition to these advantages, graduate students face several challenges as they engage in distance education. These challenges can be grouped into: preparation, communication, advisement, technical problems, and new ways of learning. The most impressive challenges were related to on-line instruction. The learning curve was extremely steep for many students, and engaging in an on-line course for the first time can be intimidating and frustrating. Several planned points of formative evaluation allowed us to identify issues early so that we could initiate immediate corrective actions and plan modifications for the future.

Adequate student *preparation* is absolutely necessary when beginning on-line courses. Many students were barely computer literate, and learning the mechanics of opening files, saving documents, posting, attaching documents, and E-mailing are basic skills prerequisite to taking any on-line course. Varying abilities with keyboarding are evident. In our early experiences the faculty did not anticipate the wide range of competencies that left many students ill-prepared. Besides computer literacy issues, students signed up for on-line courses without having adequate hardware to handle Web-based instruction. Many didn't have a modem or sufficient RAM or memory. Others didn't have phone jacks in locations near their computers. Students need detailed guidelines and orientation well in advance of beginning a Web-based course. They need information on the specifications of the computer, connecting the computer through a modem at home, and obtaining an Internet service provider. Basic computer competency skills should be required before beginning an on-line course. Finally, an orientation to the software used in the on-line courses (in our case Web-CT) is important. Otherwise, the early weeks of on-line instruction are fraught with disorganization and frustration for students and faculty.

Communication and *advisement* are major challenges for students at a distance. Many feel disconnected or intimidated by the large university, and maintaining adequate communication is essential to the success of distance learning. Distance students need personal contact with the faculty teaching their courses and their academic advisors through phone, fax, and E-mail. For those students who were less confident and self-directed, on-line education was more difficult. They wanted more frequent contact with the instructor. Many of the challenges to communication were addressed through establishing an 800 number, so that students could phone without cost to them, and creating student distribution lists for E-mail. The urgent need for rapid response is greater for distance students; therefore, faculty need to understand the isolate experience and provide responsiveness and support. Students expressed great frustration at not being able to reach faculty advisors or get quick answers to course-related questions from their faculty.

Technical problems were often frustrating for students. They complained of difficulty in accessing the server during heavy-volume times. Many were aggravated by problems with hardware and software. Without an immediate response to their situation, students risked falling behind in their course work.

The strategies used in distance education often reflect the assumptions of the emergent paradigm of learning that was discussed earlier. Graduate students have had at least 16 years of instruction in the traditional model of teaching-learning. Transferring to *new ways of learning* was often difficult. Students complained that they felt abandoned by the faculty in the course. They wanted more contact with faculty and perceived that they were cheated because they were not receiving the benefit of faculty expertise in the form of lectures or face-to-face discussions. Inadequate feedback from instructors were common comments in evaluations. In addition, students expressed real concerns that they were not "being taught" by the faculty but instead were engaged in independent study. They missed interaction with their peers and the faculty. Some commented that they wouldn't even know the people they were studying with if they passed them in the hall. Creating supportive and nurturing relationships at a distance and socializing students to a different paradigm of teaching-learning are important when beginning on-line instruction. These challenges were consistent with Reinert and Frybeck's (1997) analysis that students need structure, contact with faculty, and a sense of belonging.

Faculty Perceptions of Strengths

Faculty evaluated positively their developing comfort with the teaching strategies needed to teach interactive video, intensive, and on-line courses. When training was available from several instructional design and development professionals, the faculty learned new teaching and discussion techniques to make intensive or video courses more interesting and stimulating for students. Preparation of course materials and audiovisuals was emphasized in the training, and faculty were encouraged to learn computer-assisted methods such as PowerPoint and use of the ELMO device for switching among multiple modalities. These skills were challenging but enjoyable for the faculty as their skills and confidence developed.

A similar process was used for development of skills needed in on-line teaching. Course development required learning the specific software (WebCT), planning course content and assignments in modules, identifying and writing module and outcome competencies, and creating interesting and challenging learning activities. In the doctoral program, faculty developed a more seminar-oriented format rather than didactic instruction, with responsibility for leadership of seminars and forums placed on students. Faculty commented that this approach was evaluated positively by doctoral students and was satisfying to all. When an intensive day or two were added to the on-line doctoral courses, allowing face-to-face contact and guest speakers, both faculty and students rated the experience more positively.

Faculty acknowledged the strong potential of on-line education to facilitate access to remote students, including nurses in rural America, in urban settings across the United States and Canada, and worldwide. They viewed this option as a positive way to recruit students and also to make an impact on health care delivery and evidence-based practice in rural areas as well as developing countries. Many view the current technologies of on-line and Internet delivery as an intermediate step to full video and computer interactions when technology and infrastructure are fully available in rural America and overseas.

Faculty Challenges

Although the experiences were enjoyed by faculty, they were, however, concerned about the extensive time required for course development and implementation of all distance education models, especially on-line teaching. A strong need was indicated for more assistance in on-line or interactive course development and assistance in writing outcome competencies, as well as mentoring by other faculty with experience in on-line or interactive video teaching. In on-line courses, faculty reported spending considerable time, often at home, to read the many messages posted, engage in dialogue with individual students and groups, and evaluate projects and assignments. Faculty learned through experience how to make assignments and syllabi more realistic and feasible for the number of credits assigned. Faculty offices were not always equipped with the appropriate computers and modems to participate effectively in on-line teaching; technological glitches caused frustration more than once. The need for a strong infrastructure of support within the SON and for preparation time several months in advance of the course start date were mentioned by all faculty involved in on-line instruction.

INFRASTRUCTURE NEEDS AND ISSUES

Curriculum development resulting in curricula with a high degree of distance or remote education via differing technologies requires a strong infrastructure and overall administrative planning and support. Milstead and Nelson (1998) discussed many of these issues in depth in a recent article on preparation for on-line asynchronous doctoral courses, including preparation of technical infrastructure, administrative commitment, student services, and academic services needed for a successful program. Reinert and Fryback (1997) report that faculty must be comfortable, feel supported, and be given additional preparation time in developing on-line courses.

At the University of Colorado we learned that faculty development is absolutely essential for faculty novices to newer instructional technologies (interactive video, on-line courses, intensive classes with on-line seminars, and other strategies). Many of our faculty were fortunate to participate in several university-wide summer workshops on teaching with technology. From faculty colleagues we learned about possibilities and observed demonstrations of successful technology-supported instruction. This opportunity provided a safe and enjoyable learning environment. In addition, innovators in the SON included several faculty who boldly took risks in developing these strategies for their courses. These colleagues have become patient and knowledgeable mentors for others.

Interactive video courses require extensive resources. For example, resources on our campus included a dedicated classroom with carpeted walls and floors, good lighting, seating and table arrangements, microphones, state-of-the-art video equipment, instructional support equipment (e.g., ELMO modules), dependable communication lines, and telephone and fax capability from the classroom. Most important and facilitative of our programs was a professional technician to operate cameras and equipment and maintain a clear line with remote sites. In our case, the remote sites also had technicians. Not all universities are able to provide this assistance, but for faculty teaching in these courses, the on-site technical support made the teaching experience more professional and enjoyable. Faculty training and practice were helpful. Also important was instructional design support to assist faculty to revise courses to make video teaching interesting and engaging.

For on-line courses, the development of an Office of Informatics and a team of instructional designers and technicians is essential for supporting faculty, who possess content expertise but may be novices in technology. Sufficient planning time and scheduling well in advance of course start dates is helpful. The academic administrative team and curriculum committee of the faculty should work together to determine the delivery methods for each course during the academic year, and faculty assignments must allow for early planning and faculty development needs. Availability of updated computers with sufficient memory and speed to handle on-line instruction software and messaging and high-speed Internet connections are essential elements for faculty. Many faculty have purchased Internet service provider services at home to increase the speed and efficiency of on-line teaching off-campus.

CONCLUSIONS AND IMPLICATIONS FOR FUTURE EFFORTS

To address the technological revolution in graduate education and to promote comfort and competence of graduates using technology in practice, education, and research roles, institutions of higher education are working expeditiously to integrate emerging educational technologies and strategies. To accomplish this goal, schools of nursing with graduate education programs are exploring a variety of models and seeking expert consultations from educational technology, information services, and instructional design colleagues. Graduate students, by virtue of their age and life situations, are finding that the world of education is changing around them and challenging them to learn and use new skills and learning strategies.

Faculty, especially in more senior ranks, are also struggling to cope with a different face of graduate education. Schools that can provide a strong infrastructure and training for faculty and students will find themselves at the leading edge of innovation and creative delivery of graduate education. Possibly the most positive outcome of the use of technology in graduate nursing education is the increased accessibility of courses and degree programs to students in rural, remote, and international sites. The inclusion of these individuals will only strengthen the diversity of master's and doctorally prepared nurses but also will change the nature of health care delivery worldwide.

REFERENCES

American Association of Colleges of Nursing (AACN). (1997). *Position statement: A vision of baccalaureate and graduate nursing education: The next decade.* Washington, DC: Author.

Applebome, P. (1999). The on-line revolution is not the end of civilization as we know it—but almost. *The New York Times*, April 4, 1999.

Milstead, J. A., & Nelson, R. (1998). Preparation for an online asynchronous university doctoral course: Lessons learned. *Computers in Nursing, 16*(5), 247–258.

Reinert, B., & Fryback, P. (1997). Distance learning and nursing education. *Journal of Nursing Education, 36*, 421–427.

Siktberg, L. L., & Dillard, N. L. (1999). Technology in the nursing classroom. *Nursing and Health Care Perspectives, 20*(3), 128–133.

Skiba, D. J. (1997). Transforming nursing education to celebrate learning. *Nursing and Health Care Perspectives, 18*(3), 124–129, 148.

10

Nurse Practitioner Education: The Virginia Experience

Julie C. Novak and Cornelia A. Corbett

It is ironic that just as the time when scientific and technologic advances have prepared the U.S. health care system to make its greatest contributions to the prevention and treatment of disease, the financing and delivery problems of the system are in major discord. This chapter will present one solution to this dilemma: the effective utilization of distance education modalities through the development, implementation, and evaluation of the University of Virginia (UVA) Distance Learning Nurse Practitioner program.

THE UNIVERSITY OF VIRGINIA EXPERIENCE

The University of Virginia (UVA) PCNP data over the past 5 years support community-based education, with 59% of all NP graduates seeking and obtaining employment in rural settings and 68% of all rural students returning to their home communities to practice. For the UVA Distance Education Nurse Practitioner program, a 3-year project supported by the Division of Nursing, 100% of graduates remained in or near their home communities for completion of the master's degree in primary health care. Upon graduation, 100% accepted positions in their home communities (Novak, Obeck, & Willis, 1999). This cohort of 10 students hailed from small towns in far southwest Virginia such as Big Stone Gap, Rural Retreat, Meadowview, and Chilhowie.

Within the Commonwealth of Virginia, 68% of the 114 counties are designated as underserved. Southwestern Virginia currently has the distinction of having the highest death rate in the commonwealth. Through the use of two-way interactive video (Vtel), the UVA Distance Education Nurse Practitioner program expanded the knowledge and practice base of locally based nursing professionals without these nurses having to take extended leaves of absence or incurring a commute of 6 to 10 hours daily, 3–5 hours each way. The rural area in which the UVA's college at Wise is located is 5 hours from the main campus at Charlottesville. The area is designated as a medically underserved area (MUA) and HPSA. NPs have been well received in the area; however, NP positions offered by physicians and health care agencies often remain unfilled because of the lack of qualified applicants. The UVA School of Nursing (SON) responded to requests from individuals and a variety of institutions in offering the Primary Care Nurse Practitioner program with an emphasis on the care of the rural underserved in or near their home communities.

In charting Virginia's course for health care reform, the development of the Distance Learning Nurse Practitioner Program laid the foundation for attainment of five of the goals identified by the Virginia state legislature. Those five goals speak specifically to NP education and utilization and state, in sum, that the commonwealth shall (1) seek to train the types of professionals required by a cost-effective health care delivery system, including additional NP programs; (2) strive to remove unnecessary regulatory barriers to midlevel providers (i.e., NPs); (3) promote public/private partnerships addressing the provision of care for the medically indigent; (4) promote partnerships that recruit and train health care professionals in underserved areas of the commonwealth; and (5) promote partnerships that develop more cost-effective systems of health care delivery and financing.

Prior to the grant submission, a list of more than 100 potential students was maintained by the director of the Primary Care Nurse Practitioner program and the UVA SON Office of Student Affairs. The Southwest Higher Education Center, located in Abingdon, Virginia, maintained a list of 192 potential applicants interested in enrolling in the proposed project. Many of these bachelor's degree–prepared nurses were well known to area nursing directors, were leaders in their communities, and had already submitted application materials to the UVA Office of Student Affairs. All applicants were required to meet UVA admission criteria. These individuals had been unable to travel the 150–300 miles to Charlottesville on a regular basis for attendance in a master's or post-master's degree NP program. This collaborative effort allowed these qualified applicants to meet their educational goals while participating in preceptorships based in their rural underserved communities. In addition, Charlottesville-based students were more willing to accept distant preceptorship experiences as they were able to attend didactic classes in the distant rural location. Community and educational leaders at the distance sites confirmed their willingness to serve in an advisory capacity to the project.

Purpose

The purpose of this project was to significantly expand an existing program by adding a new education outreach site to the UVA's interactive Distance Learning Primary Care Nurse Practitioner program. Two grants from the Virginia Health Care Foundation allowed the UVA SON to increase the number of its NP faculty (Phase I) and to pilot-test the expansion of the post-master's Family Nursing Practitioner (FNP) program to two interactive VMedNet distance sites (Phase II). Seven different schools of nursing participated in various aspects of this statewide collaboration.

This proposal allowed significant expansion of this collaboration and the introduction of the master's degree program in primary health care to far southwestern Virginia in Wise and Abingdon, using distance modalities. These communities are several hours away from the nearest master's degree programs, located at Radford University in Radford, Virginia, and East Tennessee State University (ETSU). ETSU requires not only a commute but the payment of out-of-state tuition. The population of students at the northern Virginia distance site allowed a diverse applicant pool to enroll in the UVA interactive VMedNet program in Falls Church, Virginia. This distant site provides the opportunity for a clinical preceptorship exchange between UVA students and Howard University NP students. Students can request placements in rural, underserved settings in northwest Virginia or inner-city rotations with an underserved population in Washington, DC. This relationship provides a culturally diverse, mutually enriching experience for all collaborators, as UVA students have the opportunity to participate in a preceptorship exchange with placement in inner-city Washington, DC. Howard University NP students based in Washington, DC, have the opportunity to request a rural placement for a portion of their preceptorship. In addition, students from distance sites attended an educational conference and hands-on clinical workshops on topics such as microscopy, casting/splinting, and suturing/wound care on UVA grounds twice each semester.

Faculty Resources

Those who teach advanced practice nursing should be current practitioners of what they teach. Faculty and student contact should be for the purpose of communicating learning needs as well as areas of needed improvement and equivalent didactic and clinical experiences (Cook & Manly, 1996). Resources available for implementation of this project include 17 PCNPs on the UVA SON faculty, with over 100 years of combined experience. Eleven are directly involved with the didactic and/or clinical component of the PCNP program. These individuals teach the didactic component of the program to the distance sites. All of the faculty maintain an active clinical practice ranging from 10% to 60% of their time. Faculty who live and work in the distance sites are based in the distance classrooms for didactic classes, teach hands-on labs such as advanced health assessment, arrange clinical preceptorship placements, and visit each student twice each semester in his or her clinical setting. All UVA resources are available to all distance site UVA PCNP students. Accommodations are made for distance students who desire to come to Charlottesville for direct utilization of resources. Electronic mail accounts are provided for all students on admission to facilitate effective and frequent communication with the faculty and fellow students.

Clinical Resources

The UVA Medical Center, Hospital West, and Kluge Children's Rehabilitation Center (KCRC) comprise a large and complex primary, secondary, and tertiary care teaching facility. The Primary Care Center, located adjacent to the main hospital, includes more than 130 examining and consultant rooms, which provide internal medicine, family practice, pediatric, oncology, dermatology, oral surgery/dentistry, and obstetrics and gynecologic services. Hospital West offers additional clinics. In all, there are 40 outpatient clinics throughout the entire medical complex, providing more than 400,000 patient visits annually. As a regional medical center, the Health

Sciences Center serves a diverse group of patients whose health care needs are complex. The varied medical sites provide a rich range of initial experiences for PCNP students. Telemedicine capabilities link resources in Charlottesville to clinical sites throughout the commonwealth.

Clinical preceptorship sites are selected through collaborative discussions between students and course professors and are based on an assessment of the facility's ability to provide learning experiences facilitating the achievement of course and student objectives. The UVA PCNP program currently maintains formal contracts with more than 200 clinical agencies. Each area of specialization utilizes clinical facilities that provide access to populations appropriate for the specific clinical specialty, family or pediatric. Clinical experiences take place in both urban and rural health care settings, with a special emphasis on underserved rural populations.

Seventy percent of the NP clinical practice sites are located in rural settings. Those located in Charlottesville and Albemarle County also provide health care to at-risk and disadvantaged populations. Among these are two new federally funded nursing clinics operated by the SON at public housing sites in Charlottesville: Crescent Halls, a high-rise complex for the elderly and disabled, and Westhaven Apartments, composed mainly of young women and children.

The NP programs at UVA work closely with the various regional Area Health Education Centers (AHECs) to develop and support new clinical sites in rural and underserved areas of Virginia. The regional AHECs also have provided housing and travel support for Charlottesville-based students, who gain clinical experience in distant sites. As a result of this collaboration during the past 3 years, more than 45 new clinical sites have been opened, and 17 PCNP graduates have been employed in the sites where they have completed their clinical preceptorship rotation.

THE DISTANCE NP CURRICULUM

The master's degree in primary health care with a Pediatric Nurse Practitioner (PNP) or Family Nurse Practitioner (FNP) specialization was designed to reflect national health care trends and to prepare primary care experts to meet current and future needs of a dynamic health care delivery system. Sharp (1999) contends that three specific areas will have an impact on the future of NPs: communications and information technology, education via electronic technology, and quality assurance of professional skills through continued competence.

The core of the UVA distance learning NP program emphasizes technology as an intervention and as a teaching-learning modality as it weaves through the theoretical underpinnings of advanced nursing practice and research. The health policy, epidemiology, and health informatics courses prepare the graduate to function in an interdisciplinary, ever-changing health care arena. The specialty core of nutrition, advanced health assessment, pathophysiology, and pharmacology further provide a foundation for the primary care seminars and preceptorship placements that define the specialty. The applicant chooses to specialize as either a family or a pediatric NP.

Clinical preceptorship sites are assigned on the basis of optimal learning experiences, student requests, and availability. To develop experience in rural health care with underserved populations, students are assigned to at least one preceptorship site distant from Charlottesville and Albemarle County. Distance students based in far southwest and northern Virginia will remain in or near their home communities for didactic classes and clinical preceptorship rotations.

The academic and clinical content of the program is provided by a multidisciplinary, collaborative team of health care professionals. Primary care content in the curriculum includes health promotion and disease prevention, common acute and chronic health problems, women's health, well child, acute and chronic pediatric care, elder care, emergency care, and mental health problems, including substance abuse, eating disorders, depression, and family violence. Culturally sensitive community-based care is emphasized. Each course emphasizes the cultural and ethnic differences within the patient population. Strong supporting science courses, such as pathophysiology, epidemiology, and pharmacology, prepare the PCNP for the complex nature of primary care and also allow graduates to meet national and state requirements for certification and prescriptive privileges.

The core masters in primary health care courses is transmitted through VTel interactive video. Three seminars focusing on health promotion, disease prevention, common acute episodic illness, and chronic illness are part of the regular NP curriculum. They are transmitted simultaneously through the VTelNet system to the distance sites, allowing interactive learning. The pharmacology course and the didactic portion of the advanced health assessment course are also transmitted through distance learning methods. The VTel modality is supplemented with Web-based learning, audiovisual tapes, and electronic mail. The project director is in weekly communication with the distance site coordinators and the distance-based students.

This 56-credit-hour curriculum leads to the master's degree in primary health care nursing with specialization as a pediatric or family NP. These courses are completed in four semesters and a 12-week summer session of full-time study. The post-master's primary care program is designed to provide the master's-prepared nurse with the necessary skills and knowledge to assume the role of a primary health care provider. This program begins in the summer with a 12-week summer session followed by two semesters during the academic year. The post-master's curriculum is identical to the last three semesters of the master's curriculum.

Education is based on scientific and humanistic approaches. These approaches foster the student's ability to think critically and promote wellness of social and cultural diversity among the community and clients. Students assume the responsibility for learning, and the faculty provide educational opportunities for knowledge and professional development.

The curriculum for the master's degree in primary health care is a blend of general master's core subjects, specialty core, clinical seminars, and clinical preceptorships. The general master's core courses are inherent to advanced practice nursing and are required by all students in the graduate program. These classes include nursing theory, research, health care policy, and epidemiology. The specialty core courses in the PCNP program include family health promotion, nutrition in health promotion, pathophysiology, health informatics, pharmacology, and advanced health assessment. Three clinical preceptorship courses are held concurrently with didactic coursework in three seminars. A minimum of 500 clinical hours is required by NP certifying bodies, with most programs exceeding 600 clinical hours. The UVA program requires 672 clinical preceptorship hours. All didactic courses are sent to distance sites via two-way interactive video (Vtel).

The master's core courses include the following:

- Theoretical Foundations of Nursing: This course is focused on advances in developing a specialized body of nursing knowledge and related theoretical constructs. Special emphasis is placed on identification of phenomena arising from the student's own professional practice in direct nursing care. The role of perspective, concept formation, and phenomena identification in theory development is studied. Analysis and critique of nursing literature and selected theoretical works are conducted.

- Research: This course provides an orientation and introduction to the statistical methods of nursing and health care research. The course provides a foundation for informed reading and application of research findings, methods, and analytical tools. Major emphasis is placed on reading and critiquing the research literature.
- Health Policy, Local to Global: This course provides an overview of policy decisions related to the organization, financing, and delivery of health care. Social, ethical, political, economic, and ideological forces shaping American and international health policy and delivery of health care are examined. Emphasis is on informed participation in policy-making processes and the impact of health care policy on professional practice and health service.
- Epidemiology and Population-Based Assessment: This course focuses on the distribution of health-related conditions in human populations and on factors influencing their distribution. Students are presented with epidemiological methods used in investigation of such conditions and factors in order to study, control, and prevent disease. Emphasis is placed on health applications of methods to improve health care service delivery and, ultimately, health.

The specialty core courses include

- Pathophysiology: This course is designed to study selected physiological and pathophysiological mechanisms in health and disease. The course focuses on physiological and pathophysiological literature and published research that contribute to an understanding of nursing and related health care problems. Application of physiological and pathophysiological mechanisms in predicting the probable effect of changes in a biological system previously at equilibrium may be incorporated into the practice of nursing and/or health care. Review sessions are conducted at the distance sites by the distance site faculty.
- Health Promotion: Individuals, Families and Communities: This course is focused on the assessment of individuals', families', and communities' health and illness across the life span. Selected theoretical models are used as a basis for developing an understanding of the specific content and process of assessment of the family unit. In

addition, theoretical and research foundations of individual, family, and community health promotion are examined. Emphasis is placed on the use of existing knowledge to guide advanced nursing practice for the promotion of individual, family, and community health.

- Nutrition in Health Promotion: This course emphasizes identification of nutritional factors that influence disease risk and recognition that lifestyle (i.e., exercise, smoking, alcohol and drug use, and nutrition) is perhaps the most important factor in determining long-term health. This course provides NPs with essential knowledge for educating individuals and groups of all ages about sound nutritional practices. Students at the distance sites present on topics such as cross-cultural nutrition with an emphasis on Appalachian populations

- Introduction to Health Informatics: This course is designed to serve as an introduction to health informatics. Students explore the nature and functions of health informatics, the current state of the science, present and future applications, and majors issues for research and development. Topics include information processing and management, decision support, computer-based patient records and information systems, standards and codes, databases, outcomes research, and the generation and management of knowledge. The focus is primarily on informatics in the delivery and management of patient care, but students also receive an overview of current developments in structural technology. The students develop a Web site on a health promotion topic as a culminating project.

- Pharmacology: This course is designed to review, expand, and update the NP student's knowledge of general pharmacology and therapeutics. The action and interaction of the most commonly used drugs in advanced clinical nursing practice settings are covered.

- Advanced Health Assessment: This course is designed to provide the NP student with advanced knowledge and health assessment skills used in the primary care setting. Focus is on acquiring, analyzing, and refining health assessment data as a basis for the development of an accurate nursing and medical problem list. Common normal variations and abnormalities characteristic of different developmental, cultural, and ethnic groups are considered throughout the course. The laboratory portion of the course allows the student to practice advanced assessment skills in a physical assessment laboratory, newborn nursery, and school setting.

The clinical didactic and preceptorship courses include

- Primary Care Seminar I: This course focuses on (1) health promotion, disease prevention, and health supervision for infants, children, adolescents, and their families; (2) nursing and medical management of common childhood illnesses; (3) reproductive health and sexuality; and (4) women's health.
- Primary Care Preceptorship I: This course emphasizes the application and didactic content covered in Primary Care Seminar I. Experiences are provided in health promotion, problem identification, and nursing and medical management of common health problems as well as client/family counseling. The course emphasizes culturally competent health care within a developmental framework. The clinical experiences foster identification and beginning development of the NP role. Direct guidance and supervision is provided by the NP preceptors and/or physicians under the overall direction of the faculty.
- Collaborative Role Development in Multidisciplinary Practice I and II: This series presents models of collaborative practice, facilitators of and barriers to effective collaboration, and positive outcomes of multidisciplinary practice. The scope of practice, credentialing, marketing, contract negotiation, and reimbursement issues are also examined. NPs and their collaborating partners from the university or the community discuss their role development and transition within this framework. Techniques for facilitating collaboration as part of the multidisciplinary team are presented.
- Primary Care Seminar II: This course focuses on the prevention and management of clients' common acute and episodic health problems. The role of the NP in primary health care is explored. Models of collaboration and referral are critically analyzed. Breakout sessions are held for specialty groups.
- Primary Care Preceptorship II: This course builds on basic concepts, principles, and skills used by NPs in the delivery of primary health care, including health promotion and risk reduction and the identification and management of a broader range of common acute health problems. Students continue to refine their assessment, management, and counseling skills in more complex situations. Role integration continues. Direct guidance and supervision are provided by physicians and the NPs at the clinical sites under the overall direction of the faculty.

- Primary Care Seminar III: The management of chronic illnesses across the life span is explored. Health maintenance and rehabilitation issues are discussed. Breakout sessions are held for specialty groups.
- Primary Care Preceptorship III: This course is a culminating experience in which rural practitioner students continue to develop the knowledge and expertise required to provide primary health care to individuals, families, and communities. Students will continue to increase their levels of responsibility for independent individual and family health care collaboration, supervision, and management. Role integration and issues affecting practice continue to be explored, with emphasis on legal/ethical issues and establishing practice arrangements. Direct guidance and supervision is provided at the clinical sites by physician and NP preceptors under the overall guidance of the faculty.
- Collaboration Role Development in Multidisciplinary Practice II: This is the second part of the course that is designed to examine conceptual models of collaborative practice, facilitators of and barriers to effective collaboration, and positive outcomes of multidisciplinary practice. A variety of topics pertinent to the student's level of role transition and role enactment are addressed, including marketing, contract negotiations, practice expectations, and government policies that are affecting today's health care system.

FUNDING AND SUSTAINABILITY

The UVA and the SON are committed to meeting the needs of underserved populations and to NP education. A competing continuation grant will be submitted to the division of nursing as the grant objectives have been met. The locally based program will continue after the expiration of the grant period, and faculty will be 100% funded by the UVA and other sources of support (e.g., clinical practice and research grants). UVA will carry the majority of faculty salaries during the project, which will help to ensure the continuity of the program. Since the distance learning modality is expensive, its continuation will depend on funding sources, not only from the UVA and collaborating institutions but also from Virginia-based foundations that have demonstrated past support. The UVA and the SON have an extremely active development program that has been successful in identifying donors for NP education in the past. These development efforts will continue during the grant period in preparation for self-sufficiency. The university's growing commitment to the use of advanced technology and innovative teaching strategies bodes well for continued support. Currently, a partnership with a variety of pharmaceutical companies is being developed. This funding partnership would support the development of a distance technology classroom within the SON. Currently, the technology classrooms in the school of engineering are used.

The UVA SON has developed a faculty practice plan over the past year, with 10 faculty currently participating. This plan will be further developed and expanded during the grant period to provide an additional source of support. Use of the VMedNet telemedicine unit is available for the provision of clinical consultation to the distance clinical sites. Telemedicine and telehealth legislation is an area of increased regulatory activity that must be followed closely by all advanced practice nurses. Teleconsultation, patient presentation, reimbursement formulas, Internet use, and lost data are only a few of the issues to be addressed in the new millennium (Sharp, 1999).

METHODOLOGY

The Virginia Health Care Foundation (VHCF) funded a 1-year pilot project, enabling the UVA PCNP program to transmit the didactic portion of its NP program to students via distance learning at Shenandoah and Radford Universities. A multimedia network system (VMedNet) linked UVA to the Roanoke Learning Center in Roanoke, Virginia, attended by students from Radford, and the Northern Virginia Learning Center in Fairfax, Virginia, attended by students from Shenandoah University. These participants completed the program in 1997, the objectives of the project were met, and the funding ended.

The Distance Learning Nurse Practitioner Education Program was built on the VHCF-funded pilot program and collaborative projects and systems within the Commonwealth of Virginia. The focus remained on outlying rural and underserved areas. Using distance learning technology, the PCNP program was projected to two collaborative distance learning sites. In addition to its use of innovative technology to offer advanced nursing education to remote sites, the program was unique in that it serves as a link between rural and urban underserved settings. UVA's PCNP program is offered to students at one rural site in Abingdon, far southwestern Virginia, and one urban site in Northern Virginia.

Table 10.1 shows a detailed plan of action for each objective by project year, including activities necessary to accomplish the stated subobjectives and evaluation strategies.

PRAGMATICS OF USING DISTANCE MODALITIES

Faculty members should set aside 1–2 hours to meet with the distance technicians, to get to know them, to tour the facility, to learn about the equipment, and to practice using the technology. All teaching materials should be prepared in advance, and faculty should arrive at the classroom site 15–30 minutes before going on camera. The producer or engineer will be busy setting up and testing equipment during the 15 minutes before class starts. Any technical problem encountered during those 15 minutes must be solved before the class/program begins.

Teaching at a distance is highly collaborative work. It is important that the classroom personnel know the speaker's plans and expectations. The course syllabus should be provided to the assigned producer or engineer prior to the beginning of the semester. It is important to have each class or presentation planned well in advance. The plan should then be discussed with the operating engineer (Brenneman, 1998).

It is the responsibility of the speaker to ensure that all students at all sites feel engaged in the presentation. This requires the presenter to be attentive to the students physically located in the same room and those that are connected via television (Vtel). Initially, paying attention to the camera and the students located in the same room is overwhelming. Without the faculty member's attention to remote sites, however, students will often feel isolated and disconnected from the learning environment. It is important to include the remote-site students in the discussion and specifically address students at the remote site so that they are aware of your presence and interest in their input. Verbally communicate directly with the remote sites before moving forward to new material in the presentation (Brenneman, 1998).

THE ELECTRONIC CLASSROOM

Teaching in the electronic classroom offers a wide variety of options, which many faculty find exciting. These include the opportunity for elec-

TABLE 10.1   Plan of Action for Each Project Year

Methodology/Process	Evaluation/Outcomes
YEAR 01 (1997–1998)	

I   Increase access to UVA primary care nurse practitioner (PCNP) program in targeted areas.

Develop outreach programs of the masters/postmasters curriculum to two distance sites via two-way interactive video telecommunication.

Methodology/Process	Evaluation/Outcomes
1 Communicate with nursing leaders at distance sites to confirm readiness to begin requested program.	Program begins
2 Employ a coordinator and program support tech at UVA and a technician at each remote site.	Designated personnel employed or assigned
3 Contract with faculty.	Contracts developed, signed, and on file
4 Develop an advisory committee to guide program and ensure its relevancy at each site.	Advisory members established; members selected from each distance site
5 Establish VMedNet budget for courses to be transmitted to distance site.	Budget established
6 Contract with VMedNet, and schedule classroom and technology use.	Contract executed, classrooms reserved, bridging/transmission time booked
7 Provide VMedNet training to participating faculty.	Training scheduled for spring 1997
8 Faculty will modify class materials for distance learning modality.	Materials modified
9 Arrange for office space and equipment needs of clinical faculty at distance sites.	In-kind donation by distance sites; space provided in UVA NP office and faculty offices
10 Collaborate with personnel in each location to identify local experts and to develop local learning experiences equivalent to those offered to UVA on-campus students (such as suturing and casting, microscopy, and radiology).	Maintain and update expert data bank.

Evaluate the appropriateness of PCNP curriculum for telecommunication, using data collected during VHCF-funded pilot study:

Methodology/Process	Evaluation/Outcomes
1 Analyze student feedback at local and distance sites for all televised courses.	Feedback analyzed
2 Modify all PCNP courses for appropriateness of telecommunication.	Courses modified as needed and on file

TABLE 10.1 *(continued)*

Methodology/Process	Evaluation/Outcomes
YEAR 01 (1997–1998)	
3 Evaluate courses for content specific to Healthy People 2000 objectives.	Courses evaluated
4 Develop standard course evaluation form for each course that incorporates both standard evaluation criteria and telecommunication education.	Evaluation form developed and on file
5 Provide secretarial and technical support for faculty.	Support provided

Coordinate outreach of graduate nursing education through telecommunication.

1 Designate two permanent outreach sites: southwest VA/CVC (Clinch Valley College/SWHEC (SouthWest Higher Education Center), Northern Virginia.	Sites established
2 Prepare and implement budget for telecommunication technology.	Budget developed and implemented
3 Contract with VMedNet to broadcast program to two distance sites.	Contract developed, signed, and on file
4 Schedule courses with VMedNet.	Courses scheduled and published
5 Collaborate with personnel in each location to develop local learning experiences equivalent to those offered to UVA on campus students (e.g., suturing, casting, microscopy, and radiology).	Collaboration initiated, contracts signed and on file
6 Schedule an educational conference of experts at UVA for students from distance sites, once each semester.	Conference scheduled

Evaluate academic support resources for UVA distance students at each of the sites.

1 Collaborate with Health Sciences Library at UVA, CVC, and Howard University to evaluate academic support resources available to UVA distance students.	Resources evaluated and master list filed at SON and distance sites
2 Purchase or make available resource materials needed to supplement library materials available at distance sites.	Resource materials purchased; computer accounts at UVA established for UVA distance students

(continued)

TABLE 10.1 *(continued)*

Methodology/Process	Evaluation/Outcomes

YEAR 01 (1997–1998)

II Recruit, admit, and graduate nurses in PCNP program who are prepared to sit for national Family Nurse Practitioner (FNP) certification examination.

Develop a recruitment plan for both distance sites.

1	Collaborate with advisory committee and faculty at each distance site to develop targeted recruitment plan.	Plan developed
2	Revise current recruitment materials to reflect telecommunication education opportunities and emphasis on care of underserved rural and urban populations.	Recruitment materials revised and on file

Publicize the distance learning program in targeted areas of Virginia and in rural communities in adjacent states (i.e., eastern Tennessee and West Virginia).

1	Distribute recruitment materials to hospitals, nursing homes, schools, and community health agencies at distance sites.	Material distributed
2	Publicize the distance learning project in local and state nursing association newsletters in distance learning sites and surrounding areas. Articles and advertisements will be placed in newspapers in southwestern Virginia. Project director and distance clinical site coordinator will volunteer to speak to local nursing organizations about the new program.	Program publicized
3	Advertise the program at Virginia Council of Nurse Practitioners (VCNP) annual meeting, to each AHEC, the Virginia Rural Health Association, and other regional meetings as appropriate.	Program advertised

TABLE 10.1 *(continued)*

Methodology/Process	Evaluation/Outcomes

YEAR 01 (1997–1998)

Develop an advisement system for UVA distance students using standard and enhanced SON advisement procedures (e.g., phone, E-mail, SeeU-CMe©, VMedNet).

1	Develop a database system for all students admitted at distance sites.	Database developed
2	Collaborate with distance site faculty to establish network of advisors on site.	Collaboration initiated

Admit master's students to CVC distance site.

1	Admit a minimum of 6 and maximum of 10 NP students at Southwestern Virginia site.	Students admitted through standard UVA admissions process
2	Monitor student progress at each site.	Student database maintained

III **Expand the number of community-based student clinical practice sites for all enrolled PCNP students.**

Maintain current numbers of quality community-based clinical practice sites.

1	Identify community leaders in locations of student clinical experiences.	Community leaders identified
2	Collaborate with the community leaders to make student learning experiences optimal and mutually beneficial.	Collaboration instituted with community leaders

At least 70% of existing and new practice sites will be located in medically underserved areas.

1	Determine state and/or federal medically underserved status.	Status identified
2	Meet each semester at distance sites to maintain ongoing communication with community leaders to ensure familiarity regarding patient populations of all sites.	Communication maintained
3	Collaborate with community leaders in southwestern Virginia and Washington, DC, to identify a minimum of 20 new community-based clinical sites in underserved rural and urban communities.	Collaboration initiated and maintained

(continued)

TABLE 10.1 *(continued)*

Methodology/Process	Evaluation/Outcomes
YEAR 01 (1997–1998)	

4 Update contracts with all current sites.	Contracts updated and maintained on file
5 Identify, develop, and execute contracts with 20 new practice sites.	Contracts executed and on file at rural and urban sites and at UVA SON

Incorporate clinical practice experiences in underserved areas at both rural and urban practice sites as part of PCNP student preparation.

1 Formally incorporate into program an expectation that students will practice at both urban and rural underserved sites.	Written into program description
2 Collaborate with the community leaders to make student learning experiences mutually beneficial.	Collaboration maintained

IV Initiate clinical preceptorship exchange in which students from the northern Virginia distance site gain clinical experience in a rural underserved area and the clinical experience for Charlottesville and southwestern Virginia–based students can take place with an underserved urban population.

1 Identify students who want to participate in the exchange.	Project director and clinical site coordinator will meet with students interested in exchange.
2 Encourage Charlottesville-based students to attend didactic classes at the distance sites to increase their willingness to accept preceptorships in distant rural and urban underserved locations. Project director and clinical site coordinator will meet with students each semester to discuss advantages, including employment availability in rural settings.	Students will select VMedNet attendance option. Lodging provided by local community in collaboration with AHEC, preceptors, and local health care facilities

V Evaluate the curriculum with an emphasis on outcomes, and use this evaluative data for refinement and improvement of the curriculum.

1 Analyze student feedback at local and distance sites for all televised courses utilizing standardized forms.	Forms utilized

TABLE 10.1 *(continued)*

Methodology/Process	Evaluation/Outcomes
YEAR 01 (1997–1998)	
2 Continue to modify all courses as needed for telecommunication-based education, and provide linkages to UVA Teaching Resource Center to assist faculty in developing new course and evaluation tools.	Courses modified and new tools developed.
3 Evaluate training provided for all faculty teaching in distance program.	Utilize standardized evaluation forms.
4 Collect and analyze evaluation data that incorporate both standard evaluation criteria and telecommunication criteria.	Data analyzed and maintained
5 Provide feedback to participating faculty.	Summary/analysis of course evaluations provided to participating faculty
6 Participate in annual program evaluation and planning retreat.	Program to be held in May of each year; strategic plan for following year formulated.
7 Utilize evaluation materials for the improvement of the overall graduate nursing program and for planning future course offerings.	Reports and evaluation materials will be maintained and reviewed annually.
8 Meet annually with UVA development officers, advisory committees, community leaders, and foundation officials to plan for program maintenance after federal funding ends.	Strategic plan for funding maintenance formulated
YEARS 02 (1998–1999) and 03 (1999–2000)	
I **Increase access to UVA PCNP program for selected underserved areas of Virginia and Washington, DC.**	
Maintain distance learning programs to two distance sites via telecommunication.	
1 Maintain advisory committee to guide program and ensure its relevance at each site.	Semiannual meetings held at each distance site
2 Review VMedNet budget for courses transmitted to distance sites.	Budget reviewed

(continued)

TABLE 10.1 *(continued)*

Methodology/Process	Evaluation/Outcomes

YEARS 02 (1998–1999) and 03 (1999–2000)

3. Contract with VMedNet, and schedule classroom and technology use well in advance of course offering. — Contract executed, classrooms reserved and bridging/transmission time booked

4. Provide VMedNet training to any new NP faculty. — Schedule training if necessary.

5. Modify class materials for distance learning modality. — Continue modification and refinement.

6. Arrange for office space and equipment needs of clinical faculty at distance sites. — In-kind donation by distance sites; space provided in UVA NP office and faculty offices

7. Continue collaboration with personnel in each location to identify experts and develop local learning experiences equivalent to those offered to UVA on-campus students (e.g., suturing, casting, microscopy, and radiology). — Data bank maintained

Evaluate appropriateness of curriculum for telecommunication, using data collected during VHCF-funded pilot study and preceding year of grant.

1. Analyze student feedback at local and distance sites for televised courses. — Feedback analyzed

2. Modify courses for appropriateness of telecommunication. — Courses modified as needed and on file

3. Evaluate courses for content specific to Healthy People 2000 objectives. — Courses evaluated

4. Utilize course evaluation form for each course that incorporates both standard evaluation criteria and telecommunication education. — Data collected, analyzed, and maintained on file

5. Provide secretarial and technical support for faculty. — Support provided

Coordinate outreach of graduate nursing education through telecommunication.

1. Implement budget for telecommunication technology — Budget implemented

2. Maintain contract with VMedNet to broadcast program to distance sites. — Contract with VMedNet on file

3. Schedule courses with VMedNet. — Courses scheduled and published

TABLE 10.1 *(continued)*

Methodology/Process	Evaluation/Outcomes
YEARS 02 (1998–1999) and 03 (1999–2000)	
4 Maintain two permanent outreach sites: CVC, northern Virginia/Howard University.	Sites maintained
5 Continue collaboration with personnel in each location to develop local learning experiences equivalent to those offered to UVA on-campus students (such as suturing and casting, microscopy, and radiology).	Collaboration maintained
6 Schedule an educational conference of experts at UVA for students from distance sites, once each semester.	Conference scheduled

Recruit and admit both baccalaureate and master's-prepared nurses to primary care FNP program; graduate/prepare to sit for national certification examination.

II Continue recruitment plan for both distance sites.

1 Continue collaboration with advisory committee and faculty at distance sites to continue recruitment plan.	Collaboration ongoing
2 Review recruitment materials and modify if necessary.	Recruitment materials modified and on file

Publicize the distance learning program in targeted areas of Virginia and in rural communities of adjacent states (eastern Tennessee and West Virginia)—year 02 only.

1 Distribute recruitment materials to hospitals, nursing homes, schools, and community health agencies.	Material distributed to distance sites
2 Publicize distance learning project in local and state nursing association newsletters in distance learning sites and surrounding areas. Articles and advertisements will be placed in newspapers in southwestern Virginia. The project director and distance clinical site coordinator will volunteer to speak to local nursing organizations about the new program.	Program publicized

(continued)

TABLE 10.1 *(continued)*

Methodology/Process	Evaluation/Outcomes

YEARS 02 (1998–1999) and 03 (1999–2000)

3   Advertise program at VCNP annual meeting and to each AHEC division and other regional meetings as appropriate.

Program advertised

Develop advisement system for distance students, using standard and augmented SON advisement procedures (e.g., phone, E-mail, SeeUCMe©, VMedNet).

1   Maintain database system for all students admitted at distance sites.

Database maintained

2   Maintain network of advisors at distance sites.

Network maintained

3   Advise potential students and assist as needed with admission process.

Students receive adequate advisement

4   Evaluate advisement system.

Evaluation completed and on file

Admit post-master's students at each distance site.

1   Admit a minimum of 6 and a maximum of 10 NP students at each distance site.

Students admitted through standard UVA admissions procedures

2   Monitor student progress at each site.

Student progress monitored

Graduate students from each distance site who successfully complete national certification as an FNP.

1   In 6/99 and 6/00, graduate 6–10 students from each distance site and 20 Charlottesville-based NP students who have utilized the distance learning modality, thereby accepting rural underserved placements a greater distance from Charlottesville.

32–40 students (depending on numbers admitted) graduated on an annual basis

2   Provide materials from certifying bodies.

Every student qualifies to take national Family Nurse Practitioner certification exam.

3   Prepare students for successful completion of certification exam.

> 97% successfully pass certifying examination.

TABLE 10.1   *(continued)*

Methodology/Process	Evaluation/Outcomes

YEARS 02 (1998–1999) and 03 (1999–2000)

III **Expand the number of community-based student clinical practice sites for all enrolled PCNP students.**

Maintain current numbers of high-quality community-based clinical practice sites.

1	Maintain contracts with all current sites.	Contracts kept on file
2	Maintain contacts with community leaders in locations of student clinical experiences.	Contacts maintained
3	Collaborate with community leaders to make student learning experiences optimal and mutually beneficial.	Collaboration with community leaders cultivated and maintained

At least 70% of all practice sites will be located in medically underserved areas.

1	Maintain ongoing communication with community leaders to ensure familiarity regarding patient populations at all sites.	Communication maintained
2	Meet each semester at distance sites to maintain ongoing communication with community leaders, to ensure familiarity regarding patient population at all sites.	Communication maintained
3	Collaborate with community leaders in southwestern Virginia and Washington, DC, to identify potential new community-based sites in underserved rural and urban communities (year 02 only).	Collaboration maintained

tronic field trips, interesting graphics, and other visuals. The electronic classroom also offers some challenges, such as the inability to roam around the classroom while speaking and the inability to spontaneously form informal discussion circles. In general, planning ahead is critical for optimal use of an expensive yet effective teaching modality. Instead of a blackboard, speakers use an overhead camera for paper-based graphics. In some cases speakers may find the lighting distracting. The greatest challenge, however, is providing ancillary materials, such as handouts, to distance students. This most often occurs when the guest speaker does not provide handouts prior to the day of the class. Faculty are surprised at how quickly they learn to utilize the electronic options at their disposal, and working with the equipment prior to the first class "on air" experience is essential (Brenneman, 1998).

Technical Problems

The UVA Educational Technologies (ET) Department has a 99% success rate for broadcasting televised courses. Several regional UVA centers are staffed with professional satellite receive-site technicians. The staff at ET and the regional centers work together to try to solve problems quickly. Should a site miss part or all of a broadcast because of technical difficulties, a taped copy of the program is sent to the site. If a site informs the home base of problems during a course, the receive site refers to the technical sheet and calls the trouble number listed on the sheet (Brenneman, 1998).

The Presentation

When answering students' questions from the receive sites, it is important to look at the camera and to speak in a normal tone of voice. Students may interrupt at any point during class unless a specific time for questions is identified. Students should be addressed by name whenever possible, and all students at all sites should be able to hear all questions and answers. Students at the local site tend to ignore the procedures if they are not reinforced. Remind students to use the equipment as they are directed. Ordinarily, the equipment works well; however, clicks, whirrs, thumps, dial tones, and extraneous conversation may occur. It is important to ignore all of these sounds and concentrate on pertinent questions and comments (Brenneman, 1998). When there is failure of delivery equipment, faculty should continue to teach the class. Tapes are made of each class; they will be mailed to those who miss information due to technical difficulties. It is very important to end the class on time as technology requires that time be purchased on satellites or fiber lines, which are very costly. The class is cut off at the assigned time.

Instructional Design

Teaching via distance technology, like traditional teaching, is an evolutionary process. Much of what your class becomes depends on how the instruction is fashioned and presented. The teaching style coupled with the available technologies and the demographic makeup of the class are all factors that influence the course. For this reason, the design is an essential component in a distance course or program. It is through careful planning and the application of appropriate design strategies that you are best able to engage the distance learner. An ET group of professionals will help with this process. The design team works closely with the faculty to determine how to pattern course content to integrate with its delivery. This team combines the expertise of an instructional designer with the skills of a video producer, program support staff, and electronic classroom personnel (Brenneman, 1998).

Handouts

Copies of lecture notes and graphics should be sent to students prior to or at least in time for the broadcast intended. Because of the variance in equipment and hence visibility, it is always a good idea to provide students with a hard copy of detailed graphics and lecture notes. Course information can now be added to the web for students to download. Support is provided to copy and mail handouts and create Web pages. To send handouts by U.S. mail or UPS, a minimum of 5 days to copy and mail these items is required. Additional time is necessary to create a Web page and set up student accounts for retrieval of information. Interactive manuals are encouraged and enhance learning, especially in courses that require note taking, discussion, and reading.

Pictures, Charts, and Slides

Pictures and tables from books can be shown, however, under copyright laws; occasional use of these items constitutes "fair use." The operating engineer needs time to move the overhead camera in for a tight shot. Remember to use horizontal (landscape) pictures whenever possible; 35 mm slides also will have to be in the horizontal format. Let the operating engineer know the day before slides are to be used so that the equipment can be set up and calibrated.

Equipment

Personal computers (Macintosh, IBM-compatible MS-DOS) may be brought to class and connected to the video system, or software may be loaded into the MS-DOS computers. The video writer (electronic classroom) allows the speaker to highlight electronically elements of graphics, including slides or computer input. Electronic classroom personnel will demonstrate its use.

The ELMO (Vtel, videoconferencing equipment) projects graphics and overheads. It is used as a "blackboard."

Suggested Strategies

1. Specifically address questions at all sites before progressing to new material in your presentation.
2. Create a learning environment by encouraging students to interact with one another at all sites.
3. If you are providing drinks and refreshments during presentations, be sure to plan ahead and provide refreshments at all sites.
4. Make sure that students are engaged in the presentation by monitoring activities throughout the presentation.
5. Encourage the support staff to review the monitor functions with you prior to presenting.
6. Let support staff know that you will be making efforts to engage all students in the presentation and ask for their assistance.
7. Be sure to position yourself in front of the camera often so that students at remote sites can see you.
8. Wear comfortable clothes and consider layers so that you are comfortable regardless of the room temperature.
9. Avoid dark colors. Select pastel-colored shirts, tops, or blouses but avoid yellow, pink, and white.
10. Do not wear pullover sweaters that are difficult to clip the microphone to.
11. Select clothing that is subdued and simple in design. Plaids, florals, and bold stripes create screen flutter.
12. Avoid transparencies. They do not show up on the ELMO system.
13. Keep graphics to 8 1/2 × 11 inches.
14. Use blue paper under last-minute handouts and photos for which there are no hard copy or power point slides.
15. If graphics are detailed, provide handouts to *all* participants at *all* sites concurrently.
16. Select landscape orientation for all audiovisuals to fit the television screen.

17. Create graphics and audiovisuals that fill up the entire paper with 1-inch margins.
18. Use large print (no smaller than 20 font) and diagrams because the camera does not enlarge objects as a projector does (Brenneman, 1998; Novak & Wyatt, 1999).

CONCLUSION

Meeting the Healthy People 2000 and 2010 objectives requires a major shift away from the U.S. illness-oriented health system to focus on prevention and health maintenance. Nurses are the cadre of professionals who can lead the nation in this shift because of their historical emphasis on health promotion and their curricular emphasis on comprehensive, holistic, developmentally appropriate, culturally sensitive health care. The UVA Distance Learning Nurse Practitioner Program creates primary care providers who will not only meet the health care needs of both rural and inner-city populations but will assist individuals in moving toward self-care and optimal health. The program will facilitate meeting the Healthy People 2000 and 2010 objectives through direct intervention with individual and family health promotion and disease prevention activities as well as indirectly through working with communities.

REFERENCES

Brenneman, I. (1998). *Distance education faculty handbook*. University of Virginia, Division of Continuing Education, Charlottesville, VA.

Cook, S. S., & Manley, M. J. (1996). Education innovation in a time of change. *Journal of the New York Nurses Association, 27*(4), 16–20.

Novak, J., Obeck, A. K., & Willis, M. D. (1999). [Virginia nurse practitioner practice and trends: A five year longitudinal study]. Unpublished raw data.

Novak, J., & Wyatt, T. (1999). Faculty Handbook for the Use of Distance Education Modalities. Unpublished Manuscript.

Sharp, N. (1999). The road ahead for NPs. *Nurse Practitioner, 24*(2), 120–123.

11

Distance Education at the Frontier School of Midwifery and Family Nursing: From Midwives on Horseback to Midwives on the Web

Susan E. Stone, Eunice K. Ernst, and Susan D. Schaffer

We are in the midst of what has been described as the Information Revolution—the evolution from the industrial age to the information age. Many advanced practice nursing programs are just beginning to explore the opportunities available with distance learning models and asynchronous learning strategies. One nurse-midwifery education program that has been at the forefront in using a distance learning model is the Community-Based Nurse-Midwifery Education Program (CNEP) of the Frontier School of Midwifery and Family Nursing (FSMFN). This program has continued the historical tradition of the Frontier Nursing Service (FNS) by making nurse-midwifery education possible for qualified nurses in underserved and rural communities across the United States.

HISTORY OF THE FRONTIER NURSING SERVICE

The work of the FNS is legendary; it represents an important chapter in nursing history. In 1925, Mary Breckinridge introduced the use of professionally trained British nurse-midwives to the United States and established district nursing centers to provide rural Kentucky families with primary health care services. She reasoned that the health of children began with the care of the mother and that a public health nurse, prepared in midwifery, could begin care with the unborn, provide for their safe and gentle birth, and continue with teaching, care, and illness prevention throughout the life span (Breckenridge, 1981).

She located her demonstration project deep in Appalachia in rural, mountainous Leslie County, Kentucky. The area had very few roads. The midwives rode horses to make rounds, to travel to clinics, and to attend births. Mary Breckinridge felt that if this model of care could make a difference in such a remote area, then nurse-midwives could help families anywhere in the world. The success of her demonstration led to the development of educational programs to prepare additional nurse-midwives, first at Maternity Center Association (MCA) in 1932, at the FNS in 1939, and at the Catholic Maternity Center in 1943 (Rooks, 1997).

INCREASING DEMAND FOR NURSE-MIDWIVES

In the 1950s childbearing women began to awaken to the risks of routine analgesia and anesthesia and to the benefits of natural childbirth. This consumer interest, coupled with a shortage of physicians to care for women in a postwar baby boom, led to an unprecedented demand for nurse-midwifery services. Congruent with national trends in nursing education, midwifery educational programs moved into university settings, and the number of programs increased. By 1987 there were 26 nurse-midwifery education programs. Together, these programs were graduating 225 to 250 new nurse-midwives per year. However, the increasing numbers of nurse midwifery graduates were insufficient to meet the demands for midwifery services. Each issue of the American College of Nurse-Midwives newsletter carried help-wanted ads for 50 or more positions at any one time, many of them searching for several nurse-midwives to fill vacancies in one service (Maternity Center Association, 1983).

BARRIERS TO THE EDUCATION OF NURSE-MIDWIVES

Programs within university settings encountered difficulties in their efforts to expand. Limited access to clinical teaching sites, costs associated with graduate tuition, and the loss of up to 2 years of income while attending school limited student enrollments within midwifery programs. Although nurse-midwives were increasingly recruited to private obstetrical practices, as well as into hospital services, student clinical teaching experiences were limited to academic medical centers. This limited the ability of the profession to meet the growing demand for nurse-midwifery services.

The most serious constraint to the expansion of nurse-midwifery education, even today, is the availability of clinical preceptor sites. Moving nurse-midwifery education into the university centered the clinical practice in the medical model of care, competing with medical students and residents for learning experiences. In addition, the emphasis in medical education had been on the expansion of technology in all phases of perinatal care but especially in the care of women during labor. Many nurse-midwifery educators were concerned that, more and more, routine sophisticated electronic monitoring of both the woman and the fetus was serving to inhibit the development of clinical judgment and skill, which had been and continues to be the foundation of midwifery practice. At the same time there continued to be a large pool of families who did not want this "technology oriented" type of care and would opt for nurse-midwifery care, birth center care, or home birth if available (Maternity Center Association, 1983).

NURSE-MIDWIFERY AND THE BIRTH CENTER MOVEMENT

In reaction to the growing routine application of medical technology in hospital birth, women began seeking home birth with or without a midwife or doctor in attendance. Concerned about this trend, the MCA in New York City opened the first licensed freestanding birthing center in the Upper East Side of Manhattan in 1975. This birthing center provided the opportunity for women to deliver their babies in a homelike setting, free of invasive monitoring and attended by certified midwives. Birth centers have since expanded from the East Side of Manhattan to the Pacific Coast. More than any other nurse-midwifery practice setting, birth centers showcase the special skills of nurse midwives and document the importance of cooperation and collaboration between nurse-midwives, physicians, parents, public health agencies, hospitals, and ambulatory services. Birth centers interface with the health care system at all levels, utilizing nurse-midwives as primary providers and using physician specialists in obstetrics and pediatrics as consultants. Providers in these centers believe that pregnancy and birth are normal human events until proven otherwise and that informed choice, education, counseling, and time-intensive care are the essential components of a preventive health care program during pregnancy and childbirth (Pilot Community-based Nurse-Midwifery Education Program, 1989–90).

In the United States, birth centers represented a radical rethinking of the way that we provide care to healthy childbearing women and their families. At the height of the debate about whether or not any out-of-hospital birth was safe, the National Academy of Sciences Institute of Medicine appointed a committee to assess the scientific evidence on benefits and hazards of birth settings. The conclusion was that scientific evidence was lacking for all settings and research was recommended (Committee Assessing Alternative Birth Settings, 1982).

In 1985 the Hartford and Kellogg Foundations funded a 2-year prospective study of 20,000 women seeking birth center care. The report of this study, published in *The New England Journal of Medicine*, confirmed the outcomes of birth center care. Researchers concluded that "birth centers offer a safe and acceptable alternative to hospital confinement for selected pregnant women, particularly those who previously have had children, and that such care leads to relatively few cesarean sections (Rooks et al., 1989, p. 1804).

A birth center represents a place where family health is a major focus. Birth center care is midwifery care. Birth centers are designed for healthy families at low medical risk. It represents a place where nurse-midwifery practice and education can be focused. Yet it was recognized that the growth of birth centers was and is linked to the availability of nurse-midwives to staff them, which in turn depends on the expansion of educational programs and appropriate clinical practice sites.

DEVELOPMENT OF THE CNEP

The CNEP began as a cooperative effort between the MCA, the National Association of Childbearing Centers (NACC), the FSMFN, the FNS, and the Frances Payne Bolton School of Nursing, Case Western Reserve University (FPB/CWRU). These institutions share a tradition of innovation and collaboration reaching over half a century.

Nurse-midwifery leaders representing FPB, MCA, NACC, and FNS first came together first in late 1982 to explore the feasibility of a nonresidential education program to meet the needs of nurses unable to relocate to enroll in a nurse-midwifery education program. The 1983 task force was formed to begin planning for the development of the CNEP program. Members included the following individuals:

FNS—Dean FSMFN, Ruth Beeman, MPH, CNM

MCA—Director, Ruth Watson Lubic, PhD, CNM

NACC—Director, Eunice (Kitty) Ernst, MPH, CNM

FPB—Dean, Joyce J. Fitzpatrick, PhD, RN

FPB—Director, Nurse-Midwifery Program, Claire Andrews, PhD, CNM

In the fall of 1983, funds from the Department of Health and Human Services enabled the task force to begin to design such a program. Consultation was sought from Dr. Carrie Lenburg, who pioneered the New York State Regents External Degree Program in Nursing and from Dr. Cynthia France, University of North Carolina, Chapel Hill, who developed the modular design for the March of Dimes Maternal Nutrition Program. Private monies from a small grant given to FNS enabled the FSMFN and FPB faculties to meet in several working sessions to review curriculum and allocate academic credit for the completion of a master of science degree in nursing.

In 1983–85 a field trial of the CNEP concept was carried out by Ruth Beeman at FSMFN with two nurses in Arizona. Modules were sent to those two students for independent study prior to coming to the Hyden campus for 1 month of testing and intensive classroom instruction. A three-way contract between the FSMFN, a birth center in Phoenix, and a CNM-perinatologist team providing tertiary experience allowed the two students to meet all their clinical requirements without leaving their homes. Both returned to the Hyden campus for final seminars, the comprehensive school exam, and graduation with the class completing the traditional program. Both graduates did well on the American College of Nurse-Midwives (ACNM) exam and have continued to be active in the Phoenix community.

In 1985 a proposal was submitted by the MCA the Pew Memorial Charitable Trust for funds to develop curriculum materials for a nonresidential educational program in nurse-midwifery. The design of the program, now known as the CNEP, was completed in 1988. A new grant was awarded to the MCA in the fall of 1988 to begin implementation of the program on January 1, 1989 (Pilot-based Nurse-Midwifery Education Program, 1989–90).

PURPOSES OF CNEP

The primary purposes of CNEP are twofold: to provide high quality education for nurses desiring to enter the profession of nurse-midwifery and to expand the opportunities for that education in an effort to meet the increasing demand for nurse-midwives in all types of practice settings. Specifically the purposes are:

- To reduce the barriers to nurse-midwifery education.
- To meet the professional standards for nurse-midwifery practice, including specific preparation for management and operation of a freestanding birthing center.
- To increase the number of nurse-midwives prepared to practice in the birth center setting and other nurse-midwifery services to meet the projected demands for staffing.
- To contain the cost of education by including a large segment of supervised off-campus, independent study and, where possible, a work-study arrangement for clinical practice learning in a birth center.
- To prepare nurse-midwifery staff in birth centers and other practice sites to serve as faculty in the clinical instruction of students (Pilot Community-based Nurse-Midwifery Education Program, 1989–90).

DESCRIPTION OF CNEP

The CNEP is a nurse-midwifery education program designed to offer an innovative educational program to increase the number of practicing nurse-midwives with an emphasis on birth center practice. The goal is educational preparation of students through alternative pathways that are nonresidential and community-based.

The CNEP was founded and developed on the following beliefs. Nurse-midwifery provides the path for safe and thoughtful childbearing experiences, wherein choices and control reside within the family. The art and science of nurse-midwifery evolves from a solid base of knowledge and skills acquired through a combination of study, observation, and experiences. It encompasses all aspects of childbearing, beginning with conception, continuing through labor and birth to postpartum and the primary health care of women of all ages. As an art, nurse-midwifery is the conscious bending of scientific principles with creative imagination. Grounded in the scientific discipline of nursing, the practice of nurse-midwifery is humanistic, caring, and holistic in approach (Pilot Community-based Nurse-Midwifery Education Program, 1989–90).

As a nonresidential community-based program, CNEP is further based on beliefs that

- There is a large pool of nurses interested in becoming nurse-midwives if the educational program would not involve uprooting their families and discontinuing their employment.
- Learning professional skills and responsibilities is enhanced through a clearly defined program of study implemented by master professional preceptors.
- Adult learners are self-motivated, drawing on multiple experiences that may not fit traditional learning structures.
- Community-based education meets the needs of those learners for whom conventional nurse-midwifery residential programs are not available.
- The faculty-student relationship is a reflection of the CNM-client relationship in that it consists of mutual respect, responsibility, and growth (Pilot Community-based Nurse-Midwifery Education Program, 1989–90).

A "midwifery program without walls," CNEP is a 2-year, self-directed, modular course. The educational philosophy of the program assumes that the student and the faculty are partners in a common enterprise and that the student is an adult who brings to the learning process all the accumulated knowledge and experiences of life (Pilot Community-based Nurse-Midwifery Education Program, 1989–90).

Midwifery Bound

Students come to the FSMFN campus in Hyden, Kentucky, for a 5-day orientation called Midwifery Bound at the beginning of the program.

During this session, students are tested to determine their learning style and are taught to use this information to analyze problems that may occur in their progression through the program and with their preceptor relationships. Students are taught how to set up their work spaces at home and develop their own set of rules, boundaries, and timelines to assist them in planning their course of study. In addition, students spend time getting to know each other, the faculty, and how to use the computer communication system.

The Curriculum

After the 5-day orientation, the students go home to begin a period of concentrated study that takes an average of 1 year. The CNEP curriculum draws heavily from the Mastery Learning Curriculum initially developed at the University of Mississippi and implemented by virtually every nurse-midwifery education program in the United States. It is designed to meet the ACNM core competencies. It attempts to draw on the learning experiences and opportunities that abound within the students' community. It prepares graduates for a public health, community, family-centered, and business oriented approach to nurse-midwifery practice. The curriculum is structured so that students progress through several levels of learning at their own pace. The curriculum is divided into modules that specify objectives that must be mastered in order to achieve competency in nurse-midwifery. These modules are written by faculty and are continuously updated and revised. During this time of intensive didactic study, students communicate frequently with their classmates and the course faculty, often by the CNEP bulletin board system called the Banyan Tree and also by telephone.

The program is divided into four levels. Students progress sequentially through the program completing Level 1 sequences before moving to Level 2, then Level 3 and Level 4. Level 1 is designed to develop the scientific and conceptual basis for advanced practice. It provides a strand for the assessment of the individual, family, and community. It contains courses such as communication, health promotion, birth center, and reproductive physiology.

Level 2 develops the theory base for clinical practice. There is emphasis on the cognitive level of knowledge and comprehension of clinical content. It contains courses such as normal antepartum care, normal intrapartum care, and pharmacology for nurse-midwives.

Level 3 is the second period of on-site time at the school in Hyden, Kentucky. This is a 2-week intensive course with a focus on the testing and development of critical psychomotor skills and group process to begin cognitive levels of application and analysis. Students at this level perform physical examinations on each other, practice their skills on models, discuss ethical dilemmas, and present cases for group discussion. Upon completion of this level, students return to their communities to begin the actual clinical practicum with their clinical midwife preceptors.

During Level 4, students care for clients under the supervision of a qualified preceptor. In addition they are expected to complete didactic courses related mostly to clinical skills and health complications.

Depending on several factors such as prior experience, ability to spend concentrated time and effort on the program, ability to stop other work, and family responsibilities, students require between 18 and 30 months to complete the program. The average time is 24 months. Time limits for each level have been developed, and students risk dismissal if continuous progress is not demonstrated.

The Process

The modular curriculum is delivered by mail and contained in bound books. Journal articles are also supplied to the students as it is recognized that many of these students live in remote areas where they have limited access to academic libraries containing the most up-to-date literature related to nurse-midwifery. Other resources supplied to the students include videotapes, audiotapes, and CD-ROMs. Students order their textbooks from on-line bookstores. They complete written assignments and upload them via E-mail to faculty members, who grade them and send them back in the same manner. Each course has its own forum on the Banyon Tree bulletin board system. Many assignments require the student to communicate with other students via these course forums. Assignments such as presentation and discussion of case studies lend themselves very well to this asynchronous mode of learning. Students can post their assignments in the forum and then return at their own scheduled time to view the responses and add to discussions.

Exams

Each student identifies an exam proctor in her community. This is often her CNM preceptor but may be a local nurse-administrator. The proctors write letters to the CNEP stating that they are willing to assure the security of all CNEP exams and are willing to act as proctor to the student. When a student is ready for an exam, she makes an appointment with her proctor. The student then notifies the school, and the exam is sent to the proctor. After the exam is completed, the proctor mails the exam to the responsible course faculty. As students complete courses, course faculty send grade sheets to the CNEP registrar. Throughout the program, the student is continuously evaluated through written learning activities, completed bulletin board assignments, and proctored exams.

Electronic Bulletin Board

One of the exciting innovations in communication used by CNEP has been the introduction and use of an electronic bulletin board. Over 500 students and faculty are "networked" through this medium, sending public and private messages to each other, transferring file documents, and publishing bulletins of newsworthy events particularly interesting for nurse-midwives. Each course has a forum area where focused discussions take place, including student assignments such as case presentations and discussions of ethical issues. This is also an area where instructors can make announcements, address frequently asked questions, and monitor the students' thought processes as they learn to think critically. Students have their own private forum area where they can discuss issues without faculty input; faculty also have a private area. Quarterly faculty meetings are run on-line asynchronously, allowing full participation from faculty. The curriculum committee is run as a forum where faculty members can exchange curriculum documents for peer review and feedback. The faculty recently developed a process for running a faculty meeting according to *Robert's Rules of Order* in an on-line forum. This method of "conferencing" is clearly cost-effective and strengthens the teaching/learning process between faculty and students.

Course Faculty

Course faculty are nurse-midwife educators who work out of home offices. The role of the faculty is to indicate resources to be used in achieving the course objectives and to guide and evaluate the student through the learning process. Faculty live in their home communities. There are currently faculty members located across the United States from Oregon and California to Florida, Michigan, and Maine. Faculty hold regular office hours so that students can call for discussion and help. Each course has a course coordinator and, depending on the course workload, may have additional course faculty and teaching associates. The course coordinator is responsible for assuring that the course meets all objectives and is revised on an ongoing basis. Course faculty assist the course coordinator with course development and also teach by phone, computer, or on site, as well as grading papers. There is an education director who is responsible for the overall integrity of the theoretical content and design of the curriculum.

Director of Student Affairs

Three faculty members hold the title of Director of Student Affairs (DSA). Each covers a separate region of the country. One of their primary responsibilities is to provide counseling and support to students. They contact students on a regular basis to assess their progress through the program. They assist the student in problem solving, setting up learning plans with the student if deemed necessary or sometimes just listening as the student resolves her own dilemma. This support can be critical to the success of students working at a distance. The DSAs also serve as facilitators to the Regional Clinical Coordinators (RCCs) and the preceptors. They sit on the administrative team to assist in program management and evaluation.

CLINICAL EDUCATION AT A DISTANCE

One of the motivators to develop the CNEP program was the desire to be able to utilize nurse-midwives working in their own communities to provide clinical education to CNEP students. How could this be done while assuring a quality education?

A known factor was that there was a pool of certified nurse-midwives working in clinical positions all over the United States. The ACNM gathers the information regarding practicing nurse-midwives on an ongoing basis. Such information was easily attained through this organization. A second known factor was that the basic education that these nurse-midwives had attained was essentially the same. All had attended nursing programs and were registered nurses. All had then attended midwifery education programs accredited by the American Certification Council (ACC) of the ACNM. This assured that all were educated according to the standards of practice and the core competencies of nurse-midwifery as defined by the ACNM and ACC. This pool of certified nurse-midwives was considered the potential clinical teachers for the CNEP students. A complex system was developed to recruit preceptors and establish a system of checks and balances that would assure that the student received a clinical education that allowed her or him to attain competency in all clinical skills. The system worked in the beginning and remains essentially the same today.

All applicants to the CNEP are told that they must find CNMs who would be willing to be preceptors. If an interest in precepting is expressed, a CNEP program faculty member contacts the CNM and arranges to go to the site and do a preclinical site visit.

Assuring Quality in Clinical Education at a Distance

During the preclinical site visit, the regional clinical coordinator explains the responsibilities of the preceptor, reviews patient charts and practice agreements, and generally does a quality assurance review of the site to assure that it meets the needs of a student nurse-midwife and meets the standards of the CNEP. In addition, the RCC explains the role and expectations of CNEP preceptor to the potential preceptor.

If the site does meet standards, a contract between the site and the CNEP is developed. This contract explains the responsibilities of the site, the preceptor, and the CNEP. It also explains the malpractice insurance carried by the CNEP for its students and ensures that the preceptor site also carries adequate insurance.

CNEP preceptors attend a 2-day workshop on the skills of precepting nurse-midwifery students. Even though the process of teaching is included in great depth in the background of nurses and nurse-midwives, it was felt that the focus on teaching clinical skills to student nurse-midwives would be greatly beneficial. This workshop presents such topics as adult learner characteristics, learning styles, teaching styles, theories of learning, and case studies of different situations to assist the preceptors in developing their skills as clinical teachers. During the time that this workshop was required, over 1,000 certified nurse-midwives attended. Requests for offering this workshop at a distance triggered the development of a modular course for preceptors. This course can be completed at the preceptor's own pace with no travel required. It has received very positive evaluations.

The Role of the Clinical Preceptor

Clinical preceptors contract with the CNEP to provide the clinical education of the students. The preceptor is the cornerstone of the educational process. As a group, they become ad hoc faculty for the CNEP and are reimbursed for their efforts. They teach all the clinical skills required by the core competencies. The student comes to them with a very basic core set of skills, such as performing a physical exam and suturing. The preceptor builds on this knowledge and actually teaches the student all of the clinical skills necessary to practice as a certified nurse-midwife. The student carries a list of skills required. At the beginning of each clinical session the student and preceptor review what has been accomplished and develop a plan for the day. At the end of the day, an assessment is made of what was accomplished, and a plan for future goals is developed. The student's average time at a clinical site is 6–9 months. All students must complete, at a minimum, the following set of clinical experiences:

40 new antepartum visits

140 return antepartum visits

40 labor management experiences

40 deliveries

80 postpartum visits

40 newborn assessments

80 postpartum/family planning/gynecologic visits

If, upon completion of the clinical experiences, the preceptor, the student, and the RCC feel sure that the student has attained competency in all required skills, a Declaration of Safety is signed and sent to the CNEP central office. The statement declares that the preceptor "has observed the student's clinical practice and is satisfied that the student is a safe, beginning level practitioner." If the either the RCC or the preceptor or the student feels that the student needs more practice at a certain skill, the student will remain at the site until competency is attained. The CNEP currently has contracts with over 600 clinical sites located in every region of the United States.

The Role of the Regional Clinical Coordinator

As the CNEP continued to grow, it became obvious that the core program faculty could not continue to provide all site visits and contact with the preceptors that was needed. A new position, called regional clinical coordinator (RCC), was developed. Expert nurse-midwives were recruited from strategic areas in the country. This role includes many important tasks: completing the face-to-face interview with all applicants to the program, advising applicants about the availability and suitability of clinical sites, and advising the preceptors regarding the nuts and bolts of excellent clinical precepting. In addition, RCCs are counselors to the students during their clinical experience. They call students every 2 weeks during their clinical experience to review progress and discuss any concerns. They also call the preceptors every 2 weeks to assure that things are going as planned from the preceptor's perspective.

A major role of the RCC is to complete all clinical site visits. RCCs do a preclinical site visit to assure that it is a good site for teaching. In addition, they do at least one site visit during the time that the student is in the site. The responsibilities during this visit include observing preceptor/student interactions, conducting a chart review to assure that policies are being carried out as documented in practice agreements and to review the students' progress in all clinical skills. The RCC is also a problem solver and may go to the site to identify issues if there are identified problems between the site and the student. During their clinical experience, students collate daily evaluation forms that are completed with the preceptors and send them to the RCC at the end of each month for review. The RCC will use these to evaluate the student's progress and to focus their next phone discussion with the student and the preceptor.

Quality Assurance Officer

As the CNEP program expanded and increasing numbers of students entered clinical training, it became necessary to add a quality assurance officer to manage contracts with participating agencies and to validate appropriateness of the clinical sites. In a program in which the community is the setting for clinical education, the identification and aggressive management of potential and actual "risks" is critical. Although the RCCs manage the educational outcomes for the student, it became necessary to implement a corresponding administrative structure. The quality assurance officer acts as a risk management specialist, adapting accepted quality assurance procedures to the program. This specialist designs a system of contract management and maintains that system so that it is current and reflects changing protocols and standards of practice at each clinical site. The quality assurance officer examines and validates the credentials of each clinical preceptor and also provides a link between administration, faculty, and legal counsel.

PROGRAM EVALUATION

CNEP is fully accredited by the ACNM and licensed by the Kentucky Council of Higher Education. Accreditation requires strict adherence to quality indicators. There are many ongoing evaluations built in to the program. Every student must fill out a course evaluation form in order to complete the course and receive a grade. These evaluations are batched and returned to the course coordinator with no student names attached. These evaluations are used to revise and improve courses each year.

The students evaluate Midwifery Bound and Level-3 on-site experiences. Faculty review all evaluations and make changes and adjustments as indicated. When a faculty member does teach on-site at Level 3, another faculty member sits in and evaluates teaching skills. Each faculty member must recruit another faculty member for skills peer review on an annual basis. As mentioned previously, the on-line curriculum committee reviews all revisions of each course and gives feedback to the course developer.

Whenever an RCC does a site visit, she leaves an evaluation form with the preceptor to evaluate the RCC and give suggestions. These are returned to the director of student affairs of that region, and feedback is given to the RCC. Students provide a written evaluation of their preceptors at the end of the experience. The RCCs provide feedback to the preceptors.

All students are sent evaluation forms after program completion that are intended to provide an overall program evaluation. This evaluation is shared with all faculty and program staff.

One important indicator of quality is CNEP students results on the national certifying exam for nurse-midwives. Ninety-three percent of CNEP graduates pass this exam the first time. The CNEP recently completed a survey of its graduates as well as their employers. All the data have not yet been collated; this will be published in a future article. The CNEP has now graduated over 700 nurse-midwives since the first graduating class in 1991. These graduates are bringing nurse-midwifery to areas that were not previously served by nurse-midwives. Preliminary data show that greater than 30% of CNEP graduates are serving in medically underserved areas.

CNEP TODAY AND THE FUTURE

The CNEP continues to be very successful at graduating caring, competent nurse-midwives. There are currently 225 nurses in the program. Thirty-five faculty members work to provide a quality education to these students. During 1998 we published our CNEP Web site at www.midwives.org. This Web site is used to deliver information about the program. It also houses the Banyan Tree bulletin board course. Students can download this course and the software from the World Wide Web and sign on to the bulletin board as soon as they are enrolled. In addition, premier events are published and announced here. The site stores the student handbook as well as the Midwifery Bound manual. Students share their first birth stories at this Web site. In June 1999 we will publish our first credit-bearing courses on this Web site. We expect to move entirely away from paper delivery of courses over the next 18 months. We are very excited about our past success and our future plans. One of the most exciting programs currently in the development phase is the Family Nurse Practitioner (FNP) program modeled after CNEP.

The First FNP Program

The FNS originally initiated a certificate program coordinating family nursing and nurse-midwifery in a 1-year primary care nursing program in June 1970. This was the first FNP program in the United States. The initial program was divided into three trimesters. During the first trimester, all students were taught diagnosis and management of common health problems, family health assessment, counseling, and utilization of community resources. Second-trimester students had basic midwifery (prenatal, postpartum, child care, and family planning). During the third trimester, students had the option of focusing on advanced midwifery (intrapartum and newborn care) or outpost nursing (community health, district management, family dynamics, and therapy). A fourth trimester in community nursing was added in 1973. The certificate program in family nursing was offered to registered nurses with associate degree preparation, diploma preparation, baccalaureate preparation, and master's degree preparation. The program permitted nurses with all levels of preparation to enter the program in part because the school's Primex Grant (1971–72) required that primary care training be provided to all registered nurses without discrimination.

Growing Pains and Outcomes

Although formal university affiliations were sought by FNS for the development of a master's-level program, such affiliations proved to be elusive. Universities found it difficult to grant academic credit for a program offered off-campus by another agency (Isaacs, 1973). Eventually, an affiliation was developed between FNS and the College of Nursing at University of Kentucky to allow students who met graduate admission requirements to take their primary care courses at the FNS for university credit. Students were also required to take one semester of graduate credits at the University of Kentucky campus in order to complete a master's degree (Isaacs, 1973). By 1989, there were 212 graduates of the Family Nurse Midwife Program (completing both specialties) and 71 who had completed only the nurse practitioner portion of the program. Because of problems with coordinating scheduling between the two programs and concern about the work required to complete the master's degree, only 10 nurse practitioner students completed requirements for a master's degree under the agreement with University of Kentucky.

The End and the New Beginning

Difficulties with finding sufficient FNP clinical sites, faculty attrition, and concerns that a master's degree would be required for FNP programs led to closure of the FNP program in 1989. But the FNP program was not forgotten. With implementation of the highly successful distance learning program for nurse midwives and the successful affiliation with the Frances Payne Bolton School of Nursing at Case Western University, the FSMFN became interested in restarting an FNP program using distance methodology. With an affirmative feasibility study written by Nancy Fishwick (University of Maine Rural FNP program) and the endorsement of the FSMFN board of directors, planning for the new FNP program began.

Program Planning

Preliminary work to identify course writers and an FNP program director was accomplished by direct mail recruitment to FNP programs and by recruiting at national conferences. Program development for the Community-based Family Nurse Practitioner Program (CFNP) began in January 1997. Subsequent phone conferences and meetings were held during 1997 and 1998, to develop course descriptions and identify course writers. The finalized curriculum was 60 credits (similar to the CNEP) and required students to complete most of the didactic course work before beginning clinical experiences.

Shaping the New FNP Curriculum

Because the midwifery program produced graduates that were successful in certification and in practice and who had strong affective ties to the school, efforts were made to mirror CNEP teaching strategies in the CFNP program. The intensive time spent in Hyden at the beginning of the program, the sharing of frontier nursing history, the opportunities for students to share their own stories, and the maintenance of student traditions (stringing bead necklaces) served to stimulate student feelings of affiliation. Requirements that students regularly visit student forums and faculty on the Banyan Tree Computer Communication system served to keep student travelers along the self-paced learning highway from losing their way. Faculty ensure that students are competent in psychomotor skills with a second intensive on-campus session at Level 3 after students have completed most of the didactic courses. This intensive session also permits relationship building between students and between students and faculty. The credentialing and paying of clinical community preceptors was also adopted as a mechanism of ensuring control over the clinical courses. The CNEP's success in incorporating the Internet as an integral part of the program led to the decision to place all of the FNP program's courses on the Internet (www.frontierfnp.org).

CONCLUSION

The Frontier School of Midwifery and Family Nursing is very proud of its ability to provide distance education opportunities. Most of the students we serve would have been unable to continue their education without this type of program. The distance model of offering advanced practice education to nurses across this country allows the Frontier School to continue to strive to fulfill the mission and provide quality health care to "wide neighborhoods."

REFERENCES

Breckenridge, B. (1981). *Wide neighborhoods: A story of the Frontier Nursing Service.* Lexington: University Press of Kentucky.

Committee on Assessing Alternative Birth Settings, Institute of Medicine. (1982). *Research issues in the assessment of birth settings: Report of a study.* Washington, DC: National Academy Press.

Isaacs, G. (1973). The family nurse and primary health care in rural areas. *Journal of Nurse-Midwifery, 18*(3), 4–12.

Maternity Center Association. (1983). The next fifty years of nurse-midwifery education. New York: Author.

Pilot Community-based Nurse-Midwifery Education Program of the Frontier School of Midwifery and Family Nursing in Affiliation with Case Western Reserve University, Frances Payne Bolton School of Nursing. (1989–90). *Student handbook.* Cleveland, OH: CWRU.

Rooks, J. P. (1997). *Midwifery and childbirth in America.* Philadelphia: Temple University Press.

Rooks, J., Weatherbee, N., Ernst, E., Stapleton, S., Rosen, D., & Rosenfield, A. (1989). Outcomes of care in birth centers. *New England Journal of Medicine, 321,* 1804–1811.

12

Supervision of RN Distance Learning Students: The Experience of Vanderbilt's RN Bridge Program

Carolyn J. Bess

The characteristics of registered nurse (RN) students that necessitate distance education approaches include social role commitments and adult learner attributes. RNs are working adults who fulfill family roles, such as spouse and parent (Gomez, Ehrenberger, Murray, & King, 1998). RNs have identified the need for flexibility in scheduling and location of educational programs (Krawczyk, 1997). Distinctive adult learner characteristics that support the use of distance learning as an educational methodology include (a) desires independence, (b) exhibits self-motivation, (c) values relevancy of new knowledge and skill, and (d) responds positively to active learning. Distance learning provides an environment to foster independence/autonomy that is desired by the adult learner (Cravener, 1999; Gomez et al., 1998). Self-directed learning by identification of ones' own learning needs and objectives is supported by distance learning methodology (Billings, 1997; Penney, Gibbons, & Busby, 1996). In many distance learning offerings, the facilitation of collaborative learning events is evident. The participants create their own content (Cragg, 1994). The adult learner responds best when new knowledge and skills are associated with prior learning. Application of RNs' problem-solving skills to new knowledge and skills is an effective reinforcer of learning. The distance learning process promotes an active learner (Carlton, Ryan, & Siktberg, 1998; Cravener, 1999).

Distance education programs have been reported to increase RN student enrollment in BSN programs (Gomez et al., 1998). As the trend to offer distance learning courses at institutions of higher education escalates, a paradigm shift is occurring that supports the use of the Internet for content delivery and processing (Carlton et al., 1998; Cravener, 1999).

With this higher education paradigm shift in mind, the faculty of a nontraditional graduate nursing program decided to redesign the educational methodology for RN students. The RN student (admitted after completing 72 hours of prerequisite course work) was expected to meet objectives equivalent to a BSN program at the end of the first year of a 2-year graduate program. The purpose of redesigning the current instructional methodology was to increase RN student enrollment while maintaining the educational quality and rigor of the program. The goal was to weave and blend traditional and nontraditional approaches to increase flexibility related to time and location of the educational offerings. The synchronous or face-to-face interaction between teachers and students was altered by scheduling 4–5-day block classes approximately 3 to 4 times during a traditional 14-week semester. A variety of asynchronous formats were used. These formats included videotapes, E-mail, on-line conferencing, and student-selected, faculty-approved preceptors or agencies at the student's location.

INTEGRATED SYNCHRONOUS AND ASYNCHRONOUS INSTRUCTIONAL DESIGN

In the first semester, full-time RN students were expected to complete three required courses and an elective course for a total of 12 semester credit hours. The one clinical course offered in this semester focused on basic health assessment content and skills. The didactic and lab component was completed in one concentrated 4-day block of time. The lab practical was taken on the fifth day. Seventy clinical hours were spent with advanced practice nurses or physician preceptors who were selected by the student and approved by the faculty. E-mail and/or phone communication was used for addressing student and/or preceptor questions. The students were required to submit two complete history and physical write-ups on patients (due dates at midterm and end of semester). History and physical write-ups and instructor feedback comments were exchanged with faculty members electronically (fax) or through mail. The comprehensive final multiple choice exam was taken in conjunction with one of the block class sessions before the end of the semester. Midterm and final clinical performance evaluation feedback forms were submitted by fax or mail.

The second required course in the first semester fostered critical thinking, lifelong learning, and professional role development. This 3-hour didactic course used a block lecture format spread throughout the semester. Because of the focus of this course, the face-to-face, instructor-to-student contact allowed for professional socialization, role modeling, and mentoring that has been reported as deficient in distance learning methodologies (Milstead & Nelson, 1998; Penney et al., 1996). Use of a journal-writing learning activity focused on developing critical thinking abilities throughout the entire semester. The use of E-mail for faculty and student interaction and student-to-student interaction was encouraged. Evaluation strategies employed in this course were a role paper assignment, critical thinking journal activity, and oral presentation on an issue important to nursing practice.

The third 3-hour didactic course taken during the first semester focused on population-based health care principles of prevention, health maintenance, and health promotion. The videotape of traditional lecture content was used for this course because over 100 other students were enrolled in the same course. The videotaping required more precise planning related to course schedule, technician availability, and backup plans. Some audiovisual aides required more preparation time with this course. In addition, contingency plans were needed when videos were not received as scheduled by mail (Cravener, 1999). On-line conferencing was used for questions and answers related to lecture content. Separate student on-line chat rooms were available on request for student work group discussions. Evaluation methodology employed was a multiple choice midterm examination given during block course class days. A poster presentation and paper were submitted at the end of the semester.

Elective course offerings were available in a variety of formats each semester. Also, independent study options were possible, depending on student and faculty interest.

The second semester consisted of four required courses and one elective. The clinical course required 140 hours of clinical work, with a focus on the family in the community. Clinical hours were spent at self-selected, faculty-approved agencies located in the student's community (e.g., hospices and family shelters). Daily clinical logs and two family analyses were required. A written independent, family-focused proposal and project were completed. E-mail communication for questions and answers and project feedback and approval was instituted. A midterm and final clinical performance evaluation feedback form was submitted for fax or mail by the student's agency preceptor.

A 2-hour seminar course focused on the relationship of critical thinking, problem solving, nursing process, and decision making when planning care and identifying clinical outcomes. This course used a block format three times during the semester for 4 days in each block. Case studies with tutorials were used as teaching tools. Between block classes, E-mail was used for faculty and student interaction. Individual student-led case study presentations and written therapeutic treatment plans were used to evaluate student learning.

A 1-hour seminar class addressed selected topics foundational to the students' practice role. This course used a 50% block class format, meeting three times during the semester. The intent was to continue the professional role socialization process begun the previous semester and to continue to facilitate role modeling and mentoring. The other 50% of the course was on-line conferencing with faculty and student leadership and participation. On-line conference setups included forums for course announcements, questions and answers, and six topic areas. Faculty-led forum topics were ethical considerations related to rights, responsibilities, and health care and ethical issues related to death and dying. Student-led forum topics were Patricia Benner's model, collaborative practice model, mentoring, and credentialing/certification process.

On-line chat rooms were available to each student leadership group to allow for discussion and planning for student-led forums. On-line student responses were evaluated as to quantity and quality. The frequency of interactions were recorded without regard to quality. Quantity and quality were evaluated overall using the criteria in Table 12.1. The quality of student contributions were evaluated for each of the forums. Numerical scores representing quantity and quality were assigned for each student's participation in the forum. Quantity was represented by a simple count of postings. Quality was represented by A = 4, B = 3, C = 2, and F = 0–1, based on the overall criteria. Increased frequency and quality of student interactions were found with on-line conferencing. This characteristic of on-line conferencing has also been identified by Carlton et al. (1998).

TABLE 12.1 Conferencing Participation Criteria

Grade	Criteria
A	Participates in all forums by making relevant comments and posing knowledgeable questions in reaction to material posted. Reads all the required readings, indicated by relevant interactions. Maintains a professional manner in all interactions with participants.
B	Participates in all but one forum by making relevant comments and asking topic-centered general questions in reaction to materials posted. Reads most of the required readings, indicated by staying on discussion topics when interacting. Maintains a professional manner in all interactions with participants.
C	Participates in all but two forums by making general comments and asking vague questions in reaction to material posted. Reads some of the required readings, indicated by inability to consistently stay on discussion topics when interacting. Maintains a professional manner in all interactions with participants.
F	Participates in four or less forums by making general comments and asking vague questions in reaction to materials posted. Reads required readings inconsistently, indicated by inability to interact meaningfully on discussion topics. Maintains a professional manner in most interactions.

Students were expected to carry out leadership forum responsibilities. Groups composed of three students were assigned leadership responsibilities (see Table 12.2). Each student was evaluated on his or her individual leadership contributions to their forum in the areas of organization, completeness, relevancy, evidence-based interactions, and communication style. An additional evaluation strategy employed was a written ethical case study analysis submitted by fax or mail.

The last required course of the second semester addressed health care systems and related issues. This didactic course used videotape of traditional lecture format. E-mail communication to answer questions was implemented. Two multiple choice examinations were administered, one in conjunction with block classes and one take-home examination submitted by mail. Three required written projects, related to content on managed care, continuous improvement, and legal/ethical issues, were submitted by mail.

The final semester of the first-year curriculum changes has not been implemented to date. It is anticipated that similar educational methodology will be employed in the final semester. The blending of a variety of

TABLE 12.2   On-line Conferencing Student Leadership Responsibilities

Student	Responsibilities
1	To set the stage for the conference, this student posts a provocative opening statement introducing the conference topic/model. In the same forum thread, the student provides the participants a list of the forum's student leadership. This opening statement and leadership list should be posted on the first day of the 2-week forum. In addition to the introduction responsibilities, this student posts a forum summary at the end, identifying the major points covered during the 2-week forum. This summary statement should include major questions posed, significant comments made, and relevant areas explored by the participants and leadership during the forum. Summary statements are posted in the appropriate thread on the last day of the forum.
2	Using the required reference(s) and at least one additional reference, this student posts in the appropriate forum thread an outline of major areas to be discussed. Also, this student summarizes and posts significant concepts and ideas taken from the additional reference on the first day of the 2-week forum block. References are documented using APA format.
3	This student moderates the discussion by commenting on the other students' contributions and points out key concepts and ideas relevant to the topic/model discussion. To fulfill these responsibilities, the student must log onto the conference site and interact with the forum participants at least every other day during the 2-week conference period. This interaction should prompt participants' discussion by asking relevant questions to expand the discussion.

synchronous and asynchronous instructional strategies is providing RN students with flexibility related to time and location of their education.

IMPLEMENTATION ISSUES

Changing instructional methodology required preplanning to coordinate administrative support services (Milstead & Nelson, 1998). Services such as registration were handled by mail or telephone. The nursing registrar's willingness to be flexible and the established procedure of student notification of registration deadlines by E-mail were essential. Student advisement was accomplished by a combination of phone, E-mail, and face-to-face appointments during block time segments. Although multiple communication methods were chosen by individual students, the most satisfying approach noted by this writer was the practice of setting individual short appointments during the last block dates of the semester. These 15–20-minute appointments addressed the student's view of how her or his program of study was progressing.

Support services, such as student orientation to the university and school of nursing community, was a 2 1/2-day segment attached to the first block class days. In addition to the standard student orientation, the distance student needed additional assistance related to computer technology and accessing library resources electronically. Basic computer technical resource requirements provided by the school's computer technology specialists were mailed to students as soon as they preregistered. This information was provided even to prospective students on request. Ongoing computer technical support was provided by the director of the Instructional Media Center and technically competent assistants. Technology problems experienced by students were related to difficulty in installing and using hardware and software and encountering server downtime and busy peak user times. The students found the technical support responsive, but their ability to identify the nature of a problem and communicate it successfully to the technical staff was problematic. As reported in the literature, we found that provision for a technology support system to help distance students when problems occur was an essential component of a distance learning program (Cragg, 1994; Milstead & Nelson, 1998).

Library services have presented a challenge. Librarians schedule appointments for groups of students to learn search skills during the orientation days. Distance students used on-line library databases and on-campus library resources during block class segments. Students who were resourceful found additional library services available in their own communities. Textbook availability was an issue related to timing. A block class segment was usually scheduled within the first week of classes. Students purchased textbooks and class packs at that time. Assigning required readings for the first block segment was problematic. Students could not complete all the reading assignments before class. Providing access to textbooks by mail and publishing textbook requirements and reading assignments for students 1 month prior to the first block class were identified as possible solutions. These administrative services are key to providing a supportive educational environment for the distance student. Preplanning and coordinating these services were essential to the program's success.

An equally important aspect of a distance education program is the time and support provided to faculty members participating in this change in instructional methodology. Implementing a blend of synchronous and asynchronous instructional strategies has advantages and disadvantages. A disadvantage of using multiple technology approaches is based on the unfamiliarity of faculty and students in the application of technology to the learning process. As Milstead and Nelson (1998) recommended, we used a team effort to address this issue. The faculty members had specialists related to computer technology available for consultation, a multimedia production specialist was contracted for videotaping components, and faculty colleagues with a special interest in distributed learning were available to help plan on-line conferencing activities. A newly formed Center for Distributive Learning addresses issues related to all distance learning components of the program.

Advantages and disadvantages of the faculty role changes required were numerous. Faculty liked the increased flexibility of time scheduling but found the block class format a challenge to organize multiple learning activities to stimulate and motivate the learner. Faculty and students both liked the increased accessibility of faculty. E-mail and on-line conferences provided the capability to readily access faculty. As identified by Billings (1997) and Cravener (1999), there was an increase in faculty workload. More time was required for needed preplanning activities and team coordination. Faculty members needed to be involved in and informed of technology problems that adversely affected planned learning activities. If the server was down and the students did not post their assignments on time, then the faculty member needed to know. Maintaining an alertness to actual and potential electronic problems that might affect the learning event were new skills for many faculty.

Additional faculty time was needed to write messages, in contrast to in-class verbal interactions. Interactions in class are limited by time, but E-mail and/or conference postings are not limited by time and in many instances not limited in volume (pages). The increase in volume of communication and increase in multiple thoughts being expressed in one student interaction require extra faculty time to process communication and organize a response. Changes in interpersonal interactions included a lack of visual and nonverbal cues when on-line communication occurred. The faculty noted that this lack tended to make interactions more impersonal and less spontaneous. Milstead and Nelson (1998) identified faculty personality characteristics that seem to counteract this tendency. These attributes were flexibility, patience, and an ability to employ a humanist on-line conversational language style. The use of block classes also helped to offset this impersonal tendency and loss of spontaneity.

Changes in volume, pattern, and style of faculty-to-student and student-to-faculty interactions changed the faculty role. As identified by Cravener (1999), faculty surrender control to learners and move to a facilitator-of-learning role when using on-line conferencing. When using a blend of synchronous and asynchronous instructional strategies, faculty members had to be flexible risk takers.

As students adapted to a different learning environment, student role changes were identified. Using a variety of instructional methodologies required the learners to be flexible. Students in most instances were learning new computer skills. As with any distance learning format, there is an increased responsibility placed on the learner (Billings, 1997; Gomez et al., 1998). Emotional and interpersonal issues play a part in the student's adjustment to the autonomous distance learner role. Students struggled with the sense of isolation that can occur with distance learning (Carlton et al., 1998; Cragg, 1994), and the faculty used strategies to reduce the learners' feeling of isolation. Students have an increased need to develop and use their local resources, such as preceptors and agencies. There are different types of demands made on student personal support systems, such as family, friends, employers, and fellow students. Students' written and verbal communication skills were challenged by distance methodologies. Communications were expected to be concise and condensed, as well as organized, relevant, and evidence-based. Individual personalities and interpersonal dynamics had an impact on the quality of communications whether synchronous or asynchronous.

As with any group of students, variations in learning styles were expected. Providing a variety of instructional methodologies appeared to address this area of faculty concerns. The major concern was that using on-line conferencing and written assignments alone would be relying too heavily on the written word.

Another anticipated area of faculty concern in distance learning programs is providing opportunities for professional socialization (Milstead & Nelson, 1998). On-line conferencing was set up to foster faculty-monitored group interaction. Chat rooms were made available to encourage student-to-student interactions. Planned synchronous class meetings were planned in block formats. Both a question-and-answer forum and E-mail were monitored closely by course faculty members.

The clinical experience environment, when established at a distance, added to the student's responsibilities. The distance students were expected to initiate setting up a preceptor or agency about 2 to 3 months in advance of the beginning of the semester. The students were sent a copy of the preceptor role and student responsibilities for the clinical experience. Student performance criteria detailing the expected behaviors were communicated in writing. The student talked with the faculty member in charge to discuss potential appropriate sites. The student then contacted a preceptor or agency and discussed his or her interest in working with the preceptor or agency. If the preceptor or agency was interested, the student communicated that interest to the faculty member in charge of the course. If the site selected by the student was approved, the faculty member would initiate the contract process. A separate contract office exists in the school to assure coordination of clinical sites and standardization of records. Faculty members were available by phone during all steps in this process, to answer questions from students and potential preceptors and expedite the process.

To ensure the instructional quality of the distance program, faculty sought both formative and summative evaluations. Student group debriefings were held face to face in the last block class segment of each semester. Standard university course and instructor evaluations were administered at the end of every course. In the on-line conferencing course, a "fast" feedback form was used at midterm to identify what was going well or not going well. A student survey was sent by mail from the associate dean's office at the end of each semester of study. The survey form addressed student satisfaction and suggestions concerning the student's program of studies and educational methodologies employed.

SUMMARY

The redesign and implementation of an RN program to allow for distance learning was described. Instructional strategies to blend synchronous and asynchronous formats were employed. Two semesters of a 3-semester component were described, including each course focus, educational methodology, and evaluation strategies. Educational methodology implemented included traditional lecture and seminar classes, delivered in 4–5-day block classes three to four times during a semester, and asynchronous formats, including videotapes, E-mail, on-line conferencing, and student-selected, faculty-approved preceptors/agencies. Major distance learning implementation issues discussed were preplanning essentials, technology challenges, faculty role changes, student role changes, clinical experience environment, and evaluating instructional quality. The purpose of redesign was to increase RN student enrollment while maintaining the educational quality of the program. Implementation of the program is still in process, but preliminary evaluations are positive.

REFERENCES

Billings, D. M. (1997). Issues in teaching and learning at a distance: Changing roles and responsibilities of administrators, faculty, and students. *Computers in Nursing, 15*(2), 69–70.

Carlton, K. H., Ryan, M. E., & Siktberg, L. L. (1998). Designing courses for the Internet: A conceptual approach. *Nurse Educator, 23*(3), 45–50.

Cragg, C. E. (1994). Distance learning through computer conferences. *Nurse Educator, 19*(2), 10–14.

Cravener, P. A. (1999). Faculty experiences with providing online courses: Thorns among the roses. *Computers in Nursing, 17*(1), 42–47.

Gomez, E. G., Ehrenberger, H., Murray, P. J., & King, C. R. (1998). The impact of the national information infrastructure on distance education and the changing role of the nurse. *Oncology Nursing Forum, 25*(10), 16–20.

Krawczyk, R. (1997). Returning to school: Ten considerations in choosing a BSN program. *Journal of Continuing Education in Nursing, 28*(1), 32–38.

Milstead, J. A., & Nelson, R. (1998). Preparation for an online asynchronous university doctoral course: Lessons learned. *Computers in Nursing, 16*(5), 247–258.

Penney, N. E., Gibbons, B., & Busby, A. (1996). Partners in distance learning: Project outreach. *Journal of Nursing Administration, 26*(7/8), 27–36.

13

A Model for Development of a Web-based Trauma Course

Joan E. King, Jerry Murley, Sarah K. Hutchison, Judith Sweeney, and Jeanne M. Novotny

PHASE I: PRELIMINARY NEEDS AND MARKET ANALYSIS

The ongoing advances in both medicine and nursing are a double-edged sword. As we are able to provide better care to patients, especially in the arena of trauma, patients are surviving injuries that previously were fatal. However, to remain abreast of the latest advances and research findings, there is a tremendous amount of new information to disseminate and learn. Although the challenge of staying up to date with these advances can be problematic for individual care providers, it provides a fertile field for the development and implementation of Web-based computer courses. This was the very challenge that faced the Trauma Unit at Vanderbilt University Medical Center and the Vanderbilt University School of Nursing.

Vanderbilt University Medical Center is a Level 1 trauma facility with a newly opened 14-bed intensive care unit, a 7-bed observation unit, and a 10-bed stepdown unit. The unit has 63 RN staff nurses, 5 advanced practice nurses, who function in a role similar to that of a nurse practitioner, and 25 care partners or technician roles. As the unit opened in August 1998, a new staff was selected to join the unit. The staff was selected from RNs who were part of the Surgical Intensive Care Unit and also included nurses who were newly hired into the Trauma Unit or who requested a transfer from another unit within the medical center. The result was a new staff with increased learning needs, as well as an experienced staff that needed to be up to date concerning the medical and nursing standards of care to be implemented in the new trauma unit. One of the initial needs identified was the pathophysiology and standards of care for trauma patients suffering from hypothermia. The challenge emerged as to how to educate a variety of individuals with varying backgrounds and educational levels and do so in a cost-efficient manner without jeopardizing either the daily running of the unit or patient care. The answer was Web-based instruction.

At the same time, the ongoing needs of an Acute Care Nurse Practitioner (ACNP) program at Vanderbilt School of Nursing also surfaced. The ACNP track came into existence in 1995 with the development of a certification exam for nurse practitioners who had an acute care focus. There are currently 42 students in the ACNP track; they are allowed to subspecialize in cardiology, oncology, nephrology, cardiac, and general surgery as well as trauma. Within each subspecialty students have the opportunity to focus on the critical, acute, and chronic care problems of patients in each area.

Many of the students in the ACNP track expressed a strong interest in specializing in the care of the trauma patient. The challenge for the faculty in the ACNP track is how to meet the educational needs of each student, especially as there is a wide variability of clinical expertise among the students. Some students had experience as staff nurses with trauma patients; others had no experience but a strong desire to learn. None of the graduate students had experience as acute care nurse practitioners caring for critically ill patients. Hence, the needs of both an academic institution as well as the Trauma Unit merged into the common goal of creating interactive trauma-related modules to be accessed through the Web.

PHASE II: TEAM BUILDING

Based on the needs of the Trauma Unit, the topic selected for the first learning module was hypothermia. This topic was selected by the medical director and trauma nurse educator as a topic that is often inadequately covered in nursing programs. The selection of project team members with appropriate skills was critical. The roles required were those of project manager, content expert, instructional designer, graphic designer, database designer, and computer programmer. Team member selection was based on clinical expertise, area of practice, experience in Web-based teaching, and expertise in Web-based technology and instructional design. The final team consisted of three faculty members (one with extensive expertise in distributed learning and project management and two who taught in the ACNP program), the trauma educator, and the director of instructional technology at the School of Nursing, who had extensive knowledge and experience in graphic and instructional design that employ advanced technology for teaching adult learners.

PHASE III: IDENTIFYING THE GOALS AND DESIGNING THE FORMAT

Once convened, the first task for the newly formed project team was to identify the overall goal and individual objectives that were to guide the work. Although the initial goal of developing a module on hypothermia that could be mastered on the Web seemed straightforward to experienced teachers and trainers, group discussion led to the decision to develop a module that would not only meet the learning needs of the Trauma Unit and ACNP program at Vanderbilt but also meet the needs, on multiple levels, of similar institutions beyond Vanderbilt. Thus, it was decided that the learning module should be adaptable in order to accommodate different levels of care providers. Four levels of care providers were identified: (1) nurse practitioners, (2) graduate students, (3) staff RNs, and (4) technicians or "care partners." Although adding considerably to the complexity of content development and computer programming, this decision added capability that exceeded that of the traditional classroom.

Other objectives identified included (1) dividing the content to be taught into smaller units or subcomponents in order to facilitate learning; (2) focusing on the topic of hypothermia as it pertains to trauma patients; (3) including content on pathophysiology, assessment parameters, interventions, potential complications and protocols; (4) developing specific learner objectives for each section; (5) developing quizzes for each subcomponent; (6) developing a final exam; (7) providing immediate feedback as to the correct answers for the quizzes and final exam; (8) making it possible for participants to earn CEUs or course credit when applicable; (9) tracking detailed student performance data; (10) centrally organizing data for easy and secure retrieval by faculty managers via the Web; and (11) creating Web-based evaluation instruments to collect ongoing student suggestions for module upgrades.

To address the first objective of writing subcomponents, it was decided that even the pathophysiology content could be broken down into a number of sections, including introduction and definition of terms, the body's normal mechanisms for generating heat, coagulopathies, cardiovascular changes with hypothermia, oxygenation and respiratory alterations with hypothermia, and finally a summary of the overall physiological changes that accompany hypothermia (see Table 13.1). Each section was followed by a short quiz. Thus, by using sections to subdivide the complex patho-physiology of hypothermia into smaller units and by using the quizzes as a tool for immediate feedback to the learner, the objective of facilitating the mastery of the complex content was achieved. The same approach was used for developing the sections on assessment, interventions and protocols.

PHASE IV: DEVELOPING THE CONTENT

Once the format of subunits or sections, followed by quizzes, was decided on, a review of the literature was conducted, and key articles were selected. The trauma educator then accepted the challenge to "write" the first draft using PowerPoint™. To facilitate the work of the team, drafts of the presentation were shared via E-mail, and ongoing dialogue and suggestions were made. Thus, team meetings were kept to a minimum of one every 2 weeks for the first month and monthly thereafter. Because one of the

TABLE 13.1   **Hypothermia Module Content**

Thermal regulation
Hypothermia
Coagulopathy
Oxygenation and respiratory changes
Cardiovascular changes
Review
Assessment
Diagnostic laboratory
Planning and interventions
Protocols

major objectives was to have the module adaptable to different levels of providers, the decision was made to develop the most complex level first and then modify the content for the different levels of providers. Also, School of Nursing faculty determined that graduate students in the ACNP program would be accountable for the same information that was developed for the nurse practitioners. This meant that only three levels of content had to be written: one level of content for the nurse practitioners and graduate students, a second intermediate level for the staff RNs, and a third basic level for the technicians.

A difficult task for the project team was to decide how the modules differed between the advanced practice section and the staff RN section. The team concluded that both groups needed the same understanding of the pathophysiology and assessment parameters, but differences between the learning levels existed in the application of the content. For example, both the nurse practitioner level and the staff RN level had to know about the changes in coagulation as the result of hypothermia, as well as the cardiovascular and respiratory alterations that develop with different degrees of hypothermia. But the staff RNs' unit on assessment and their quiz focused on assessing for these changes, whereas the nurse practitioners' unit included content concerning the anticipation of specific complications and what laboratory and diagnostic tests to order. The sections for the nurse practitioners also included what interventions to order based on protocols.

For the technicians the initial decision was to select specific content within particular sections that had initially been developed for higher level learners. Thus, rather than writing a separate presentation for the technicians, their learning materials, objectives, and quiz questions were selected from those written for the staff RN and the nurse practitioner. However, during the first phase of piloting, it became evident that the content presented had to be simplified and written at a level more appropriate to the educational background of a technician. Hence, the key concepts about hypothermia and the changes it can produce in the body were presented to the technicians in a simplified form, with the overall message that these are critically ill patients, whose conditions quickly change. A section was also developed for the technicians to educate them about the types of interventions a technician might assist with. In addition, the module for the technician indicated the type of equipment and supplies that should be available for any hypothermia patient.

As the content was developed, it became evident that terminology and abbreviations were used that, if not clearly understood, could prevent learners from understanding more advanced content. These are the critical "hidden mental skills" revealed in the task analysis of instructional design (Clark, 1989). These terms and abbreviations provide a fertile field for development of future Web-based modules, lending themselves to "hyper-linking," but they also indicated a need to develop a glossary for the existing module. Following a number of team discussions, terms and diagnoses were selected, and a glossary was developed. The creation of the glossary accomplished two purposes. First, it served as a reference for participants. Second, it allowed the content writers to keep the content display screens concise and unencumbered by distracting details. Examples of items that appear in the glossary are acute respiratory distress syndrome, coagulopathy, disseminated intravascular coagulation, and left ventricular stroke index, as well as normal ranges for laboratory data such as PT and PTT. (See Table 13.2.) When the glossary was developed, a bibliographical list was compiled that would allow students to use Web-based resources, journals, and books to clarify and supplement the content presented in each section of the module.

PHASE V: DEVELOPING THE LEARNER PRACTICE AND ASSESSMENT TOOLS

Once the content was written for each section, the team focused on writing appropriate learner objectives and a practice quiz for each section. The objectives were written with the specific intent of directing each level of

TABLE 13.2 Terms Included in the Glossary

ABGs	FSP
ADH	HCT
ARDS	Hgb
Bronchorrhea	LOC
CAD	MDF
CHF	PRI
CHI	PT
CI	PTT
CO	QTI
Coagulation Cascade	Rewarming
Coagulopathy	Set-Point
DIC	SVR
EDVI	

learners to the content they should focus on while studying each section. The quizzes were used to help integrate the content taught. Many of the questions in the quizzes contained case studies that helped the learner apply the content to the clinical arena. For both the nurse practitioner and the staff RNs, many of the objectives and quiz questions were the same. But when appropriate, the nurse practitioner had more difficult questions pertaining to the anticipation of potential complications and orders that may have to be written.

After developing the hypothermia content, unit objectives, and quizzes, a final exam was developed. A case study was presented for the final exam, and the various questions focused on the level of hypothermia present, identifying appropriate anticipated pathophysiological changes, assessment findings that would follow, and finally interventions that had to be anticipated and/or implemented. For the nurse practitioners, questions were included on orders and patient care protocols. The initial final exam consisted of 11 questions but later was expanded to 14 questions for RNs and 18 questions for nurse practitioners.

PHASE VI: INSTRUCTIONAL PRINCIPLES AND TEACHING MODALITIES

As the team continued to work, it became evident that the task of developing a Web-based learning module on hypothermia was more than just writing a number of presentation screens about the pathophysiology and treatment of hypothermia. It became evident that, as educators, we had to address a number of "instructional communications" issues relating to pedagogic principles, course management and computer-user interface design (Hannum & Hansen, 1989). One issue was how to best utilize the quizzes and the final exam as learning tools within themselves. Because an objective of the team was for quizzes and the final exam to serve as learning tools themselves, the team made two decisions. The first decision was that each learner would receive immediate feedback as to whether her or his answers were correct or incorrect. The second was that feedback for each question would be accompanied by the rationale as to why the correct answer was correct. This approach was used for all the quizzes and the final exam.

To accomplish this instructional strategy, the team relied heavily on the expertise of the director of instructional technology at the School of

Nursing. The director developed a computer program that immediately scored each quiz and the final exam and then posted the answers, as well as the correct answer and the rationale for the correct response. However, in the feedback for the final exam, it was decided not to display the questions, the list of choices, and the choice of the learner so that questions could be reused as a measure of content mastery should a learner need to repeat the course. The learner's attention would be directed toward reviewing the essential content of the module rather than the score and exam.

Another issue concerning testing that the team wrestled with was whether all quiz activity should be recorded and, if so, whether scores should be incorporated into the learner's "final grade." Again, the team leaned in the direction of employing quizzes as an opportunity for learners to apply new learning and to learn by way of immediate feedback and to gauge the level of mastery they had attained. Also, the team discussed whether the learner needed to review the material and prove mastery of each unit before being allowed to proceed to new content. This led to other questions: Could learners simply take the final exam without having progressed through each section? Could learners go back over previous sections? Could they retake the quizzes and the final exam? Most of these questions arose from inquiries by the director of instructional technology, prompted by the practical need to determine programming issues before continuing with development of the courseware.

The director articulated alternatives based on his experience in computer-based instruction and his familiarity with available programming resources. As the team struggled with these issues, it was apparent that we had to put ourselves in the place of our students and see ourselves as learners who wanted to progress through tasks quickly. However, as educators we saw the need for immediate feedback where one could learn from one's mistakes. Hence, the decision was made that learners must proceed through each section sequentially and that they could not progress to the next section until they had reviewed all content and taken the appropriate quiz. Upon taking the quiz and reviewing their answers and the rationale, it was then left up to learners to decide if they needed to review the section. If a learner wished, he or she would be permitted to return to previously visited material at any time during the module and could take the quizzes as many times as needed to master the content—that is to say, until the learner took the final exam, at which time he or she would be required to reenroll, to restart the process.

Because quizzes could be taken more than once, they were not incorporated into the final grade. The final exam was developed as the ultimate evaluation of content mastery. A certificate of completion would derive from the final exam, indicating a date, content level and score. The certificate could then be used as a final documentation of competency or as a prerequisite for an exam or check-off in the presence of a proctor, instructor, or supervisor. Hence, the final exam could be taken only once, and the grade on the final exam could be determined if students had mastered the content. For RNs, nurse practitioners, and graduate students that meant that the grade on the final exam determined whether they were eligible for CEUs or class credit. A score of 85% was set as the required passing grade for either RNs or any nurse practitioner wanting to receive CEUs. After taking the module and the final exam, if the learner did not receive a grade of 85% or above, the learner would be encouraged to reenroll in the course and retake the module.

PHASE VII: DATA COLLECTION

Although the team strove to make the module on hypothermia as learner-friendly as possible and hence developed the module to provide immediate feedback and flexibility in reviewing each section, the members were also interested, from an educational perspective, in knowing who the learners were and how well each performed on each section. The team's objective was to use each learner's performance as an evaluation of how well the module was organized and written. Hence, although the learner's performance on each quiz was not incorporated into the final grade, detailed data as to how each learner performed on each section, including how many times they took each quiz, how much time they spent viewing each screen, the sequence of their movements within the module, and all their scores were recorded in a course database. In addition, learner demographic data was recorded in the database, and learners were given an opportunity to periodically update this data whenever they enrolled or reenrolled in a module. Demographic data were collected that not only allowed the team to ascertain who the learners or customers were, but it also allowed the team to determine if different types of care providers did better or worse on the module. Thus, data were collected that allowed the team to determine if new RNs, RNs with no trauma experience, or seasoned trauma care providers differed in their level of performance in each section and in the final exam. These data helped to evaluate and modify each module as needed.

Although team decisions revolved around whether the presentation screens were clear and understandable and whether the quiz and exam items where appropriate, another entire series of questions and decisions surfaced that revolved around the development of a database that would provide the data necessary to evaluate the module (1) from a core content perspective, and (2) from a program design perspective, to ensure that the courseware worked reliably, efficiently, and with ease of understanding by a variety of users. This reinforced the practical decision made early in the project to divide the work of the team into two subgroups. One group worked on developing the core content, and the second group worked on organizing the database, writing user instructions, determining possible instructional and data collection strategies given the technology, designing the computer-user interface and performing computer programming. Therefore, a dual-layered computer program were developed: On one dimension the program displays module content to the user's Web browser and guides the user through each section, quiz, and final exam. On a second dimension the computer program was developed to provide Web-accessible, interactive database support as previously described.

Because of the complexity of the work being done and with an eye on constructing an adaptive learning system that would support unsupervised student activity on multiple modules at multiple levels, it was critical for each member and each subgroup to provide timely feedback to each other. To accomplish this, the director of instructional technology placed a shell of the program design on the Web early in the project and populated it with examples that suggested paths of development. Then he implemented each section on the Web as it was written or revised so that all could visualize the product as a functioning whole. Team members were encouraged to access the course on the Web and to submit frequent and immediate feedback to other members via E-mail. This fast-track approach helped to hasten project development, as each member could better understand how all parts related and how instructional design issues differed from those encountered in the classroom and offered new learning opportunities. This not only enabled the team members to provide feedback about course content, objectives, quizzes, and exam, but it also allowed the members to determine how easy it would be for learners to negotiate the course on the Web.

This process helped the team to appreciate the need for a learning module that was user-friendly. Thus, we served as the beta testers for our own module, and it became evident that the ease with which one could navigate within the module and visually comprehend information was as important as the content being delivered. It became evident that if entering into the module was too complex or progression from section to section was confusing or time-consuming, learner interest could be lost. Also, the ease with which one could advance from screen to screen and the ability to access the glossary or bibliography and return to a specific slide were all design issues that were addressed.

PHASE VIII: THE PARALLEL DEVELOPMENT: DETAILS OF COURSEWARE AND DATABASE DESIGN

In parallel with development of the hypothermia content, the director of instructional technology and his staff began to construct a course management shell, the courseware, to register and authenticate users; to organize the overall presentation of instructional communications, including navigational and core content; and to collect and retrieve data securely and efficiently on the Web. The courseware designers created a simple but distinct graphic look and interactive feel for the program. During the first month the director attended every other content design meeting to better understand the special demands of the course concept in general and the hypothermia module in particular. Then he met as a member of the team to share insights about the instructional strategies that could be employed by drawing on available Web functions and tools.

The instructional design model employed by the team was not entirely linear. After each stage the team convened to evaluate the product to date and reflect on the design process itself. The team's primary yardstick was the needs of stakeholders in the project. This pattern of development is similar to Nadler's (1982) continual evaluation and feedback cycle, which incorporates the future stakeholders into the process in order to develop flexibility and assurance of applicability.

Database tables were created in Microsoft Access. Special Web programming tags, made possible through an application called Cold Fusion, were added to typical HTML programming tags to create dynamic, database-driven Web pages. Cold Fusion, distributed by Allaire Corporation, is an application server layer positioned between user requests of the Web server and the secure course database. In addition, the courseware subgroup wrote and illustrated detailed instructions for students about how to navigate the course and what to expect in its functionality. Without extensive real-time instructor intervention, this detailed, step-by-step guidance proved indispensable.

An essential part of the project team's strategy was the creation of an automated course that would allow students to proceed at their own pace while satisfying the need for them to master interdependent learning tasks in a prescribed sequence (Hannum & Hansen, 1989). The main Web page for the hypothermia module functioned as if it were a table of contents, hyperlinking every resource required in the module within two clicks of a user's mouse. Of practical significance to the courseware designer, the team decided to require the students to progress in a linear fashion through module content, with one topic building on the previous one. As previously stated, quizzes at the end of each section of content could not be accessed until all the previous content pages had been visited. However, learners would be permitted to review any materials as often as necessary, except for the final exam. In terms of design issues, this meant that the computer program had to guide the student's progression in a linear fashion and at the same time permit flexibility in reviewing screens or sections as often as necessary.

A student study schedule was the primary interactive guide to learners throughout the module. Every time students visited the schedule screen, the page's programming queried the database of student activity for a student's personal record and returned an up-to-date checklist of learning tasks completed or yet to be completed. The schedule, in conjunction with other small Cold Fusion programming templates, called every time pages were visited and regulated student movement throughout the module. The student study schedule, along with the learning objectives page, also provided students with an overview of the organization and relationship of all module content (Reigeluth, 1983).

PHASE IX: IMPLEMENTATION

Because a teacher was not going to be available to clarify or amplify the content on each screen, it was vitally important that each screen be clear and provide the specific content and details that would be needed to master the module. To accomplish these objectives two phases of piloting were undertaken. The first phase of piloting consisted of two faculty members and a nonnurse program developer who piloted all three levels of content. Their feedback was invaluable. As one would expect, it is frequently easy to assume that each screen is very clear and understandable and that each quiz or test item is appropriate. Because those who piloted the module had not been involved in the development of the core content or courseware, they served as unbiased evaluators. On the basis of their feedback some of the screens were rewritten to clarify important points. Also, a number of the testing items were rewritten to provide more clarity, and three new items were added to the final exam. In addition, as previously discussed, the decision was made to rewrite the module for technicians, to simplify the content and focus on the technician's responsibilities when assisting in the care of a hypothermia patient.

Once the recommendations from the initial piloting were completed, the hypothermia module was then piloted with actual staff in the Trauma Unit at Vanderbilt. Two nurse practitioners, five staff RNs, including a staff nurse who was also a graduate student in the ACNP track at Vanderbilt, and three technicians were asked to pilot the series.

In summary, the development of the hypothermia module on the Web was an interdisciplinary project. It required the combined expertise of computing, the Web, graphic and database design, and clinical and educational expertise. The development of the module really existed on two levels at once. The first level consisted of content selection, the development of content displays, and development of objectives, quizzes, and the final exam aimed at three tiers of students. The second level consisted of two layers of computer programming: one that guided learners through the Web course itself and a second program that tracked and queried data, such as the type of learner, his or her credentials and clinical experience, and his or her individual performance on each quiz and exam. This in turn provided appropriate information to the Web browser of both students' and course managers' requests. Through the integration of these two levels of work, an interactive computer learning module was created that has the ability to present new and updated content to a variety of learners in a variety of settings at any time and any place. For the student, it truly takes the "trauma" out of learning new material and remaining current in a highly specialized field.

REFERENCES

Clark, R. C. (1989). *Developing technical training: A structured approach for the development of classroom and computer-based instructional materials.* Reading, MA: Addison-Wesley.

Hannum, W. H., & Hansen, C. (1989). *Instructional systems development in large organizations.* Englewood, NJ: Educational Technology Publications.

Nadler, L. (1982). *Designing training programs: The critical events model.* Reading, MA: Addison-Wesley.

Reigeluth, C. M., & Stein, F. S. (1983). The elaboration theory of instruction. In C. M. Reigeluth (Ed.), *Instructional-design theories and models: An overview of their current status* (pp. 335–381). Hillsdale, NJ: Erlbaum.

14

An International Education Model: The Experience of the School of Nursing at the Catholic University of Chile

Ilta Lange, Mila Urrutia, Sonia Jaimovich, and Cecilia Campos

Concern for the future of the nursing profession has resulted in a movement to improve nursing education and nursing research throughout the world (Freda, 1998). Because nursing is a universal profession challenged by global issues, nurses from different countries must collaborate with each other to address common problems and develop strategies that improve health and nursing care. Nurses in an international partnership can assist in effecting change for nursing practice. International education will help nurses to understand health problems and issues globally and give them a wider perspective about the influence of political, economic, and social factors on health and health care. This wider perspective will allow them to make comparisons of leadership and labor force issues and improve health care by learning about new nursing roles that have been successful in other countries. As nursing moves to a global perspective, the schools of nursing in Latin America have to find innovative strategies to offer their students international opportunities in spite of economic, cultural, and language barriers. Educators must raise student awareness of opportunities that exist to expand knowledge and skills in health care and nursing. Global information sharing will become necessary to practice nursing effectively in the new millennium (Goldberg & Brancato, 1998; Freda, 1998), and students and faculty have to learn how to access and use this information. Today, information and ideas can move between countries rapidly, and mutual challenges and solutions can be examined, all of which adds to the potential for comparing and improving health care and nursing practice (Lee, 1997).

The School of Nursing of the Catholic University of Chile (SNCU) has participated in networking with a great number of Latin American and U.S. schools of nursing since 1983. Many of these programs have been sponsored by the W. K. Kellogg Foundation. This experience has taught us that international work can be very empowering, and it has been an effective strategy for identifying the strengths and weaknesses of the SNCU. However, the goal to develop a cost-effective and replicable international education model for faculty, students, and clinical nurse mentors was included in the strategic plan of the school.

In this chapter, successful and ongoing international activities carried out in partnership with WHO Collaborating Centers in Nursing will be described, mainly from the Chilean university perspective. These can be considered the basic components of a cost-effective international education model for faculty and students that can be longlasting in spite of local resource restrictions. This cross-cultural experience is preparing Chilean and U.S. nurses to better understand the health care needs of diverse populations, strengthen transnational nursing relationships, and broaden opportunities for international research. These experiences have increased the commitment of Chilean nurses to learn English and to consider seriously graduate studies abroad.

The first systematic international education activities were initiated in 1995, when our school received for the first time U.S. nursing students coming from three North American schools of nursing, all of which are WHO/PAHO Collaborating Centers for Nursing. These schools share characteristics that we have identified as key factors for successful and satisfying international experiences. Some of these are as follows:

- Explicit interest in Latin America.
- A horizontal approach to international collaboration, which means that this collaboration is recognized as an experience where both institutions have something important to teach and to learn.
- Recognition that the interinstitutional linkage is based on a trusting relationship, where cultural aspects are recognized and respected.

- An interest for building an ongoing partnership that will help develop the profession through collaborative education and research.

In the construction of this international, cost-effective education model we have identified the following components:

1. Visiting scholar program.
2. Short-term visiting faculty exchange.
3. Incorporation of an international component in currently offered courses.
4. Visiting professorships.
5. Invitations to nurse scholars who come to Chile for other purposes to lecture at SNCU.

VISITING SCHOLAR PROGRAM

Since 1995 the SNCU has served as an international host institution for the Minority International Research Training (MIRT) program coordinated by the College of Nursing at the University of Illinois at Chicago with the financial support of a Fogarty Grant. The purpose of the MIRT program is to provide international research experiences to minority nursing scholars, develop leaders in the field of nursing science, and increase collaboration in the resolution of global health issues.

Our school has hosted during these years, eight MIRT trainees, each for a period of 8–12 weeks. Four students came from the College of Nursing at the University of Illinois at Chicago, three from Frances Payne Bolton School of Nursing at Case Western Reserve University, and two from the College of Nursing at George Mason University. During their stay in Chile, the students participated in an ongoing research project in primary health care. Additionally, they had the opportunity to get acquainted with the Chilean health care system, observe professional nursing roles, increase their knowledge in self-care nursing and in primary health care by visiting hospitals and health care clinics. The nurses at the Catholic University of Chile have developed a self-care nursing model with the support of Kellogg Foundation, which has been replicated in various health care services in Chile and other Latin American countries.

The program provided MIRT students with an opportunity to learn about nursing and health care in Chile and broadened their frame of reference. It taught students that different countries share similar health challenges and that often the strategies used to address a problem are different because of cultural differences. The only limitation to taking full advantage of the experience was the language barrier for those students who did not speak Spanish. This limitation was partially solved by assigning a Chilean bilingual peer as a mentor for the non-Spanish-speaking students. This role fostered the interest of the Chilean bilingual peers in improving their English language proficiency. It also fostered their understanding about global nursing issues and gave them an opportunity to better understand how nurses are educated in the United States and what their role is in the health sector, in guidance of health policy, and in the community. It also helped them recognize that it is a great asset for Chilean nursing that nurses are exclusively educated at the university level. The exchange with the MIRT students increased Chilean students' interest in graduate education abroad. The linkages established through the MIRT program provide new international opportunities for faculty and students.

SHORT-TERM FACULTY VISITING SCHOLARS

In 1996 two faculty members from SNCU who had acted as preceptors for the MIRT students were invited by the College of Nursing at the University of Illinois for a 5-week visiting scholar program in the United States. The purpose was to develop a clearer understanding about the overall MIRT project, to meet faculty and deans of the institutions that had sent students to Chile, learn more about their undergraduate and graduate nursing education programs, and their international research interests, and explore international funding opportunities for future international projects. The experience was a highlight for the Chilean visiting faculty, and it was a key strategy to transform this first international contact in an ongoing international partnership with the three mentioned institutions.

In 1999, with financial support from the International Visiting Professorship Program of the Catholic University of Chile, two other faculty members from the SNCU were visiting faculty scholars at George Mason University (GMU) for a 2-week period. The purpose of the visit was to observe how the nursing curriculum has been implemented and managed in this school and how theory is linked with practice at the undergraduate level. SNCU faculty had the opportunity to attend classes and lectures and visit clinical sites. This faculty visit was carefully planned as a follow-up activity of a 3-month visiting professorship program at SNCU. In 1998 a faculty member from GMU acted as a consultant in the curriculum change process that is taking place at SNCU and in developing a strategic plan for faculty development. The impact of this visit will be appreciated in the near future, in its faculty development dimension as well as in its influence on the new curriculum. It takes time to realize and appreciate the full meaning of international experiences (Watson, 1995).

The short-term visits are a good way to learn about nursing education and health conditions in another country. They produce motivation for more international exchanges. In addition, these exchanges are very useful as orientation or consultation visits, and they help identify the need for further faculty exchanges with long-term goals. For nurses, who are mainly women, short-term visits are more feasible to carry out than exchange activities lasting several months, because of economic, family, and work responsibilities. However, they do provide an immersion process.

INCORPORATION OF AN INTERNATIONAL COMPONENT

"Seminario Profesional" and "Trends and Issues in Professional Nursing"

Since 1996, a pilot project has been carried out to promote interactive and cooperative learning experiences for undergraduate students, between SNCU and Case Western Reserve University (CWRU) Frances Payne Bolton School of Nursing. The collaboration between the two schools occurred through the course "Seminario Profesional." This course is required by all senior-year nursing students at SNCU (average, 39 students); its companion course for senior students attending CWRU is "Trends and Issues in Professional Nursing" (average, 58 students). Its goal was to create a model for global education collaboration through the use of electronic communication and information technologies. Internet resources such as E-mail and the World Wide Web were used.

Its objectives were to introduce and promote global electronic learning among students of SNCU and CWRU; to demonstrate the value of interactive, transnational education as an effective supplement or alternative

to study tours abroad; to incorporate multicultural learning into the preparation and expectations of undergraduate nursing students; and to increase
the understanding of global nursing and health problems and needs of a
culturally diverse patient population.

The dean of the Frances Payne Bolton School of Nursing, Dr. Joyce
J. Fitzpatrick, visited Chile in 1996 to inaugurate this distance learning
course, first of the kind in Chilean schools of nursing. She gave a lecture
to our students that was transmitted by videoconference to their partners
at CWRU. In this conference the participant faculty members of both
schools met each other as well as some of the students. In 1997 a second
videoconference facilitated the communication process among student
partners, who felt more at ease in writing to each other after they had
met on the screen.

During these 2 years, however, communication problems persisted,
consisting largely of language barriers and E-mail difficulties. The biggest
challenge for the success of this course was to find a strategy to maintain
communication among partner students and faculty in spite of the differing
vacation and semester schedules. This schedule discrepancy delayed assignments and produced inconsistency in the type and amount of information that students were giving and receiving. This imposed excessive stress
on the students who had to present final papers with the input obtained
from their international partners at the end of their own school semester.
The creation of an international Web site project is presently in process
to solve most of the problems that have been identified.

In spite of the difficulties encountered, those student groups at SNCU
who were able to exchange information with their U.S. partners shared
with us their view of the international component in this course. "It was
great for us to have this experience even though we had problems with
communication"; "I lost my fears about going to the U.S. to get my
master's degree" (this student is presently applying to enter the master's
degree program in a U.S. university); "I believe this course was very
important for us because we had the opportunity to share information
about nursing in Chile, practice English, and improve our computer skills,
and we met new people and learned about nursing in the United States";
"It was a great experience, which demanded lots of perseverance; it was
specially interesting to compare the nursing leadership challenges in Chile
with those in the United States. We were also surprised to learn how
different nursing education is in both countries. To meet North American
students was entertaining and informative."

As a consequence of this joint course initiative, our school received an award in 1998 to develop an Internet course for Spanish-speaking nurses, with technical support from educational television and the distance learning department of the Catholic University of Chile. This Internet course "Nursing and Self-care" will be offered for the first time in 1999.

International Research Experience for Master's Students

In 1999, Frances Payne Bolton School of Nursing at CWRU made it possible for their master's degree students to attain the research course requirements of "Inquiry III" through an international research experience. Two master's students selected the SNCU to attain this goal. They interviewed most of the nurse faculty during their 2-week stay in the country. The purpose was to identify the research questions that concerned the nursing faculty of the SNCU as a way to understand the most relevant nursing problems in Chile and to be able to facilitate future research linkages among CWRU and SNCU faculty. Through this research project they defined research goods, designed a tool for data collection, collected the data, and learned how to analyze it by using the EPIINFO statistical program. Through this process, they had the opportunity to meet nurses of all age groups and with diverse professional experiences, who shared with them their view about nursing in Chile. They also had the opportunity to visit health care facilities with students and faculty and were invited to social and family activities.

For the Chilean faculty, this was a very rewarding experience. The U.S. master's degree students helped them in clarifying their research ideas in writing abstracts in English and in obtaining bibliographical articles which were not available in the local libraries. It is expected that this study will facilitate collaborative research projects among faculty from CWRU and the SNCU. This student exchange program has been evaluated as highly successful from the perspective of students and the faculty of both schools.

International Administration Practicum for a GMU Student

During the past 4 years several international common projects have been developed between GMU and the SNCU, and each new project has opened new possibilities for international education. A new experience has been an international preceptorship to allow a student from GMU to meet the requirements of the Administration Theory and Practicum in Chile, which is her home country. To comply with the objectives of this course the student participates in the design of a clinical tutor project at the SNCU that requires the application of all her administration skills. This new international education strategy has proved highly satisfactory for the student as well as for the preceptor, because it has been an opportunity for innovation and knowledge sharing. As the student at GMU has access to full text articles through the GMU library, the process of bibliographical reviews on successful assistanceeaching models has been very efficient.

This project, which is considered a priority at the SNCU, will be concluded in a record time because of the time and effort dedicated to it by the student of GMU. This experience has been highly successful because the deans of both schools know and trust each other, and the master's student at GMU is a former student of the SNCU and therefore knows the system very well. For this reason, she needed minimal orientation to start working on her project.

INVITATIONS TO NURSE SCHOLARS TO LECTURE AT SNCU

It is not uncommon that nurse leaders are invited by health institutions, nursing associations, or other universities as consultants or seminar participants. However, there are no adequate networking mechanisms established to obtain this information in a timely manner to explore the possibility of having these scholars come to our school to offer a short workshop or to give a lecture to students and faculty.

Since 1996, the SNCU has made a systematic effort to contact in a timely manner nurse scholars who will be visiting Chile to invite them to our school. This strategy has been shown to be highly cost-effective for our school and a complementary experience for the international nurse consultant, which widens international nursing linkages and future collaborative project opportunities.

An example was the Third International Nursing Conference, which was cosponsored by the School of Nursing of the Universidad Austral in Valdivia and the Association of Chilean Schools of Nursing. A large cadre of nurse leaders attended that meeting and several were faculty members at schools of nursing with WHO/PAHO Collaborating Centers in Nursing. To get to Valdivia, all international travelers had to come to Santiago first, and therefore the possibility of having some of the international conference participants visit before or after the conference at our school was quite feasible. The SNCU organized at the school several workshops with nurse faculty members of CWRU, the University of Illinois, GMU, and the University of Texas at Galveston and invited nurses from nurses' associations and from the health care institutions where our students practice.

At the same time, activities were organized for international nurses who wanted to lengthen their visit in Chile, visit Santiago, and learn more about the country and the health care system. A 3-week traveling seminar was organized for eight African nurses who were sponsored by the W. K. Kellogg Foundation to attend the conference and learn about primary health care in Chile. Students and faculty of the SNCU had a wonderful opportunity to meet and share experiences with the African nurses and learn about nursing in Botswana, Swaziland, Lesotho, Zimbabwe, and South Africa. They also had the opportunity to participate in workshops with nurse leaders from the United States, to learn from them and help them understand the Chilean culture and health and nursing challenges in Chile. The additional efforts for the partners involved in this complementary experience were cost-effective, and philosophical commitment to international collaboration was clearly present in all parties involved.

VISITING PROFESSORSHIP

The strategies previously described have been facilitated and complemented with the yearly presence of a visiting professor. This has been made possible by the generous financial support of the Catholic University of Chile. The purpose of the visiting professor program is to offer a large number of undergraduate students an international educational experience through a course. The school of nursing learned to include continuing education, research, socialization, and consultation objectives to the visiting professorship program to increase the impact of this experience on students, clinical nurses, and faculty.

Professors from University of Illinois and GMU have acted as visiting professors in 1997 and 1998, respectively. Once back in their home institutions, networking has continued, and they have facilitated several of the projects that have been described above. Perhaps the most important asset of the visiting professorship program is the role modeling, as a teacher, researcher, clinician, or consultant. Several lessons have been learned, which will be reported elsewhere.

The opportunity to write this chapter is also a result of the international education model. We were invited to write this chapter by nurse leaders who have been our international partners since 1995. They have empowered us to share our experiences and have helped us in editing this chapter. For most Latin American nurses it is very difficult to publish in the international literature because of lack of experience and language limitations. We strongly believe that through our international work we will be able to better prepare our nursing students to work effectively in a global world, influence other schools of nursing to implement international education strategies, and continue trying out cost-containment strategies to maintain a cost-effective and replicable international nursing education model at our school of nursing that can contribute to improving nursing around the world.

REFERENCES

Freda, M. (1998). International nursing and world health: Essential knowledge for the 21st century nurse. *American Journal of Maternal Child Nursing, 23*(6), 329–332.

Goldberg, L., & Brancato, V. (1998). International education: A United Kingdom student partnership. *Nurse Educator, 23*(5), 30–34.

Lee, N. (1997). Learning from abroad: The benefits for nursing. *Journal of Nursing Management, 5*(6), 359–365.

Watson, J. (1995). A Fulbright in Sweden: Runes, academics, archetypal motifs, and other things. *Image: The Journal of Nursing Scholarship, 27*(1), 71–75.

15

The Future of Nursing Education: Marketability, Flexibility, and Innovation

Patricia Hinton Walker

At the end of the 20th century it is important to take note of where nursing has been and plan for the future. Albert Einstein said, "I never think about the future. It comes soon enough." But nursing needs not only to think about the future but to plan for it as well. We know that nursing will change in the future because we can already observe the changing roles for the professional nurse. Nursing education is changing because the future requires that nurses become autonomous leaders, as accomplished in the art and science of nursing as they are in the business of nursing. McCloskey and Grace (1997) state, "The challenge to nursing education is to make modifications that will prepare practitioners for the future rather than maintain the emphasis of the past" (p. 128). In this chapter the three primary ways that nursing is changing—competency-based education, focus on outcomes rather than process, and building partnerships— will be examined.

The role of the professional nurse is changing to that of an autonomous profession, where nurses are self-sufficient, independent caregivers rather than being employed primarily in hospitals or offices. The role of the nurses is changing so much that we don't have a clear picture of what nursing will be like in the future. This makes attracting students to the discipline one of the greatest challenges for the future. Mary Mundinger (1994) wrote, "Today, on the brink of a new millennium, scientists and policy makers recognize nursing as the health profession with the most untapped contributions for improving the health of our nation" (p. 9). We are challenged, then, to be not only educators but also public relations specialists, who must communicate this information to potential students. There is an adage familiar to many of us: nursing was born in the church and raised in the military. This paradigm has changed drastically over the years, but the impression is lasting. Our public relations mission is significant in changing perceptions about the field of professional nursing.

At the University of Colorado School of Nursing (CU-SON) we are actively working to adapt our curriculum to meet the changing role of nurses in the new millennium. While maintaining connections to its history, the faculty, staff, and administration have positioned the school as a model for survival and leadership in the new millennium. New curricula must be designed to meet the changing roles and responsibilities of nurses for theory-guided, evidence-based, reflective practice in the context of a global environment. Also, we must shift from process-oriented education to competency-based curricula designed to remove many of the barriers of traditional education through both its design across programs and its delivery methods. At the CU-SON we have engaged the assistance of Carrie B. Lenburg, EdD, FAAN, to reengineer our programs and develop faculty for competency-based, outcomes-driven education.

Another innovation at CU-SON is the development of one common conceptual framework for all four degree programs: baccalaureate, nursing doctorate (ND), master of science, and doctor of philosophy (PhD) degrees. By accepting the challenge of developing one framework, one set of outcomes (which are differentiated per program), faculty are courageously positioning the school of nursing for changes in nursing education, which will even include the futuristic BSN-PhD educational option. One competency-based curriculum across all programs also removes barriers that force students to "stop in and stop out" and encourages "customers" to achieve career goals in more creative ways instead of the lockstep learning of the past.

Our new curriculum is addressing the future through the use of four practice-inquiry foci: (1) human experience of health-illness-healing, (2) human/technology interface, (3) environmental context of health and health care delivery, and (4) quality and cost-effective outcomes. These represent a shift for the entire faculty (*SON Curriculum Redesign*, 1998). The concept of practice-inquiry focus also can be seen as a model for other schools of nursing. Other schools can identify practice-inquiry foci that are consistent with their mission, purpose, and faculty. These foci have enabled the CU-SON to focus on our strengths while building for the future. In addition, they formalize the integration of our research and practice missions with our educational programs.

Another requirement for this curriculum for the future involves the use of technology that we recognize will be increasingly significant in the future. To that end, we are working on putting all courses on the Internet in the future. Currently, we have 10 courses that are Internet-based. We are also offering courses that combine the Internet and two-way interactive video. This is going to be a significant change in the future, when nurses seeking continuing education opportunities are unable to leave their home/work environments to come to campus for classes. It is also important, on this level, that the curriculum is competency-based. To assure that nurses are receiving the necessary education, we have to formalize the way we test them for competence on many levels. CU-SON's marketable and flexible programs and continuing education offerings will ensure lifelong learning, the key to maintaining professional competence.

Finally, we wanted a curriculum that would integrate teaching, learning, and research for both students and faculty, again creating a model for other programs. The four focus areas previously cited represent modules that will guide teaching, learning, and research for everyone at CU-SON. To address the divisiveness that sometimes exists among nurses educated at different levels, students will work together across all programs on a capstone project, designed to integrate education, practice, and research. We are interested in preparing leaders in theory-guided and evidence-based practice because we believe that this is the future of the nursing profession.

Of course, there is no way to predict what the future of nursing will really look like. There was a time in our not so distant past that most nurses worked in hospitals, and we thought that would never change. McCloskey and Grace (1997) emphasize that "nurses will need to be versatile in using the [information super] highway, and knowledge will be a vital commodity for nursing personnel at all levels. An ever-expanding role for technology is to be expected, and a shift toward a global perspective will be required as the interdependency of all communities on the planet becomes increasingly apparent" (p. 137).

The future of nursing education must move toward competency-based education. The National Academy of Science tells us that to prepare leaders for the 21st century we have to teach students to be more adaptable and flexible, as well as technically proficient (McCloskey & Grace, 1997,

p. 137). A competency-based curriculum enables us to evaluate and document students' actual abilities objectively and consistently. The competency-based curriculum now used at the University of Colorado School of Nursing was developed with Carrie Lenburg's assistance and implements her Competency Outcomes and Performance Assessment (COPA) Model (Lenburg, 1999; Redman & Lenburg, 1999). The Model specifies competency outcomes for a given program, or course, and the critical elements required for each of the practice skills embedded in the performance-based competency outcome statements. Students are informed of these required competency outcomes, related skills, and critical elements from the outset of the educational program or courses to facilitate achievement of the competencies required for actual practice.

Core practice skills (competencies) include such categories as assessment and interventions, communications, critical thinking, management, leadership, human caring, teaching, and knowledge integration. These overall skills and each associated sub-skill have a set of specified critical elements that must be performed by the student to document abilities at the specified level in the course or program. They form the foundation for insuring that examiners (instructors) are objective and consistent in assessing students' actual abilities within the context of actual professional practice requirements.

For example, the skill of incorporating cultural competence in clinical practice might include the following statements: "By the end of this course, the student will be able to: 1) Show respect for diverse values and preferences of other individuals and groups; 3) Integrate knowledge of cultural variation into professional practice." Or the skill of critical thinking for case managers might include: "At the designated time, the case manager will: 1) Write the specific question to be explored, including related components; 3) Describe methods to be used, including subjects, timeline, and methods of data collection and analysis" (Lenburg, 1999). Other skills might require students to develop research questions, implement professional roles, plan nursing care for a designated client, promote cultural competence in professional practice, adapt technical procedures in a home care setting, and make clinical decisions to client-related needs and data (Lenburg, 1998).

As we look toward the next century, nursing education will have to include competency testing and evaluation. This will be critical as more and more education takes place through technology rather than face-to-face.

In addition to educational competencies, the future of nursing requires that we look at outcomes. As the profession of nursing has changed, we are moving from a process orientation to an outcomes-based orientation. Outcomes have to be evaluated in terms of cost, health status, patient satisfaction, and caring. As nurses, we are changing the way we look at our profession. We must change our focus to health promotion and disease prevention; relationship-centered care; holistic and interdisciplinary approaches to care; the mind-body relationship in care; collaboration, cooperation, and consensus in improving the health of communities; and overall community-oriented nursing to assist individuals and families in solving their own problems related to health and wellness (Lacey, 1997, p. 153).

To examine outcomes, we return to focus on the need for theory-guided, evidence-based practice. Androwich and Haas (1997) remind us that "with no paper or electronic documentation trail, justifying the value of nursing is problematic and the care rendered by nurses becomes invisible" (p. 218). As we work on defining the role and mission of nurses in the next century, we cannot allow ourselves to be invisible. We must use strategies to improve marketability and visibility, both as providers of care and in the policy arena through outcomes research.

In an environment where all nations of the world are trying to manage care in cost-effective ways, outcomes are becoming more and more important. "High-tech and high-cost care, which has traditionally been delivered in hospitals, has been reexamined, resulting in a shift from hospital-based to alternative models of community-based care" (Walker, Baker, & Chiverton, 1997, p. 37). The need for outcomes of care measurement has increased. Donabedian (1988) sets forth a framework for measuring quality, which includes three concepts: structure, process, and outcomes. Data collected by practitioners in practice and with billing records can be examined to measure cost and quality outcomes. This will assist the nursing profession in documenting the value of nurse practitioner care (Walker et al., 1997, p. 43). Nurses in practice increasingly need to focus on the relationship of cost to care.

Traditionally, the cost of nursing has been assumed into the patient's room and board in the hospital. With nursing moving out of the hospital and into community-based settings, this will have to change. "It was assumed that the care nurses provided in implementing the physician's treatment plan was going to have a positive effect on patient outcomes. Of course, little or no energy went into demonstrating that this was indeed true" (Fetter & Grindel, 1997, p. 247). Nurses are now expected, with good reason, to show that nursing interventions directly result in desired patient outcomes. Fetter and Grindel (1997) argue that the Nursing Minimum Data Set will enable us to document nursing diagnoses, interventions, and outcomes. Additionally, the American Nurses Association (ANA) has supported production of other nursing information systems, including the Nursing Interventions Classification, the Omaha System, and the Home Health Care Classification System. Examples of patient/client outcomes that can be measured include length of stay, satisfaction, readmissions, surgical wound infections, adverse outcomes, and waiting times, as well as many others.

Satisfaction is another outcome of care of value for study within the nursing profession. As practitioners in care environments, we must assess what we know about the quality of care we can reasonably provide in these settings. Nursing's challenge is to link "caring" to patient satisfaction. Building on Jean Watson's work at the University of Colorado, we are accepting the challenge of linking the measurement of "caring" as an outcome related to patient satisfaction.

Finally, the future of health care will require that we form partnerships with businesses, physicians, and communities. The United States currently spends almost 14% of its gross national product on health care, significantly more than any other country (Walker, 1997). Unfortunately, we in the United States cannot claim that clinical outcomes are significantly better when compared with other countries internationally. For example, regarding infant mortality, the outcomes are clearly worse.

Another future challenge for nursing education is developing partnerships. The ability to form and sustain partnerships may be one of the most important skills facing health care professionals today. We know that clinical outcomes are improved when we work in partnership with patients. Partnerships with employers, insurers, consumer groups, and government agencies will be necessary to coordinate and efficiently provide accessible health care to all people. The development of international partnerships will also bring accessible care around the globe. Creating effective partnerships can be very challenging. We must meet many goals in creating these partnerships:

1. *Work in cost-effective ways.*
2. *Focus on improving patient outcomes.* These outcomes include medical, psychological, social, and functional.
3. *Helping organizations transform healthcare delivery.* Health care organizations can create a vision, culture, and mission to transform healthcare delivery systems

from reactive to proactive organizations in order to promote patient self-care; develop comprehensive prevention programs, including behavior change; reduce unnecessary healthcare utilizations; and improve access of services to meet patients' needs.

4. *Use evidence-based methods to justify clinical practice.* Evidence-based methods influence which clinical approaches to use. These methods can guide administrators and patients to use interventions for which there is definite evidence of their effectiveness.

5. *Work in interdisciplinary ways.* Work as part of teams to provide healthcare services. Practitioners need to work together to maximize the performance of the team. This approach represents a shift from the solo practitioner to a team approach in which the primary care physician is often responsible for coordinating the delivery of healthcare in an efficient manner.

6. *Use partnership skills to empower patients and colleagues.* Empower patients and families to promote their autonomy, responsibility, and control in addressing health issues and in reducing the need for health care services. Partnership skills help patients take a greater role in self-care and preventive care and to adapt to acute diseases and adjust to illnesses more effectively; assess and manage their own psychosocial problems; take greater control over and responsibility for managing their chronic disease; improve their functional abilities; minimize dependency upon their practitioners and the healthcare system.

7. *Manage chronic diseases efficiently.* Chronic disease programs assist practitioners to enhance the quality of patient outcomes and to reduce complication rates and healthcare costs.

8. *Facilitate health behavior change effectively.* (Botelho, 1998, pp. 24–27)

We are at a crossroads in health care delivery, where creating and implementing these kinds of partnerships will be essential to the future of care.

A partnership usually refers to a legal relationship involving a close cooperation between parties with specified and joint rights and responsibilities, an alliance is an association that furthers the common interests of its members, and a consortium is a combination of members that is formed to undertake an enterprise beyond the resources of any one member (Walker, 1998). It is clear that health care providers who are willing to unlearn old paradigms of control, hierarchical relationships, and patriarchy and to learn new ways to assist organizations and communities in partnership building will be more likely to survive and be valued in a changing health care environment.

The patient-client relationship is where health care partnerships begin. This partnership must be extended to incorporate family members in providing health care. Core principles of partnership include the following:

1. Healthy mind-body split.
2. Respect culture differences.

3. There's no substitute for a good relationship.
4. Respect each other's paradigm.
5. Promote a "community of caring."
6. Adopt a population-based perspective.
7. Make families part of the health care team.
8. Develop a common mission. (Cited in Suchman, Botelho, & Walker, 1998, p. 64)

Such partnerships lead to desirable health outcomes for patients with a variety of needs.

In summary, the keys for the future in nursing education content are

1. *Leadership development.* We should be actively teaching nurses how to lead and manage.
2. *Critical thinking and problem-solving skills* will be essential for these new health care leaders. Critical thinking and problem solving also will ensure better patient care.
3. *Evidence-based practice* is the future of health care.
4. *Clinical competency in a variety of settings* will create nurses who can practice in most settings. As the focus of health care moves from hospitals to community-based care, we will need nurses who are competent in a variety of situations.
5. *Collaboration and communication* are necessary for effective delivery of care.
6. *Outcomes focus*, including cost and patient satisfaction will help guide our practice.
7. *Cultural competence* is required of all health care professional in order to communicate effectively with patients.
8. *Appreciation of research directed toward practice and educational evaluation.* If we are to develop research-guided practice, we must focus our research on those endeavors that will influence practice. We also have to constantly evaluate our educational programs that guide advanced practice.

Today, at the end of the 20th century, nursing is experiencing a renaissance. For nursing, this renaissance involves the birth of new and varied roles. In the 21st century we will be looking at new ways to market and recruit more bright young people from diverse cultures who choose the profession of nursing. We are moving from apprenticeship, one-to-one models of education, to more flexible methods; however, we cannot lose the caring and mentoring connections that make nursing education unique.

Innovations in education will naturally lead to changes in practice. These changes in practice are ever evolving but will include a reinvigorated focus on outcomes of care and building partnerships. We are very fortunate to live at a time that allows new opportunity for innovation and to see so many interesting changes in our chosen profession. Changes in delivery of care and technology must be embraced.

REFERENCES

Androwich, I. M., & Haas, S. A. (1997). Ambulatory care nursing: Concerns and challenges. In J. C. McCloskey & H. K. Grace (Eds.), *Current issues in nursing* (5th ed., pp. 216–222). St. Louis: C. V. Mosby.

Botelho, R. J. (1998). Negotiating partnerships in healthcare: Contexts and methods. In A. L. Suchman, R. J. Botelho, & P. H. Walker (Eds.), *Partnerships in healthcare: Transforming relational process* (pp. 19–49). Rochester, NY: University of Rochester Press.

Donabedian, A. (1988). The quality of care: How can it be assessed? *Journal of the American Medical Association, 260,* 1743–1748.

Fetter, M. S., & Grindel, C. G. (1997). Recent changes and current issues in medical-surgical nursing practice. In J. C. McCloskey & H. K. Grace (Eds.), *Current issues in nursing* (5th ed., pp. 243–257). St. Louis: C. V. Mosby.

Lacey, B. M. (1997). Advancing community based-community focused nursing education: Challenge for change. In J. C. McCloskey & H. K. Grace (Eds.), *Current issues in nursing* (5th ed., pp. 148–154). St. Louis: C. V. Mosby.

Lenburg, C. B. (1998). Competency-based outcomes and performance assessment. The COPA Model. Unpublished workshop materials.

Lenburg, C. B. (Sept. 30, 1999). The framework, concepts and methods of the competency outcomes and performance assessment (COPA) Model. *Online Journal of Issues in Nursing.* Available www.nursingworld.org/ojin/topic10/tpc10_2.htm.

McCloskey, J. C., & Grace, H. K. (1997). *Current issues in nursing* (5th ed.). St. Louis: C. V. Mosby.

Mundinger, M. (1994). *The Pfizer guide: Nursing career opportunities.* New York: Merritt Communications.

Redman, R., Lenburg, C. B., & Walker, P. (1999). Competency assessment: Models for development and implementation in nursing education. *Online Journal of Issues in Nursing.* Available www.nursingworld.org/ojin/topic10/tpc10_3.htm.

SON curriculum redesign: Glossary. (1998). Unpublished document, University of Colorado Health Sciences Center, School of Nursing.

Suchman, A. L., Botelho, R. J., & Walker, P. H. (Eds.). (1998). *Partnerships in healthcare: Transforming relational process.* Rochester, NY: University of Rochester Press.

Walker, P. H. (1997). Toward a comprehensive health care system: Business and provider coalitions. In J. C. McCloskey & H. K. Grace (Eds.), *Current issues in nursing* (5th ed., pp. 427–433). St. Louis: C. V. Mosby.

Walker, P. H. (1998). Community partnerships: Building collaborative models for care. In A. L. Suchman, R. J. Botelho, & P. H. Walker (Eds.), *Partnerships in healthcare: Transforming relational process* (pp. 51–61). Rochester, NY: University of Rochester Press.

Walker, P. H., Baker, J. J., & Chiverton, P. (1997). Costs of interdisciplinary practice in a school-based health center. *Outcomes Management for Nursing Practice, 2*(1), 37–44.

Index

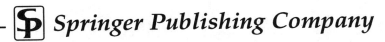
Springer Publishing Company

Telemedicine and Telehealth
Principles, Policies, Performance and Pitfalls

Adam William Darkins, MD, MPH, FRCS
Margaret Ann Cary, MD, MBA, MPH

"The most comprehensive resource on telehealth. Clearly a must read for those who feel telehealth can rebuild the physician-patient relationship."
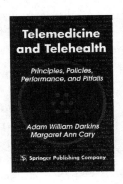
— **Charles Safran,** MD
Chief Executive Officer
Clinician Support Technology

"This is the thinking person's gateway to the world of telemedicine...these authors set the stage for nearly everyone involved in planning or evaluating a telemedicine program, policy, or research project."

— **Douglas A. Perednia,** MD
Founder and President
Association of Telemedicine Service Providers

Telemedicine and telehealth are changing the face of health care delivery and becoming a multi-billion dollar industry. The authors provide practical insights and advice on transforming telemedicine programs into successful clinical services.

Contents: Introduction • Definitions of Telemedicine and Telehealth and a History of the Remote Management of Disease • Telehealth: A Patient Perspective • Telehealth and Relationships with Physicians • Using Telehealth to Make Health Care Transactions • Telehealth Services • Regulatory, Legislative and Political Considerations in Telehealth • The Market for Telehealth Services • Contracting for Telehealth Services • The Business of Telehealth • The Management of Telehealth Services • Choosing the Right Technology for Telehealth • Other Important Influences on Health Care that Affect the Future of Telehealth • References • Glossary of Terms and Abbreviations

2000   328pp.   0-8261-1302-8   hard   www.springerpub.com

536 Broadway, New York, NY 10012-3955 • (212) 431-4370 • Fax (212) 941-7842